Praise for *The End of Alzheimer's*

"*The End of Alzheimer's* is a monumental work. Dr. Bredesen completely recontextualizes this devastating condition away from a mysterious and unsolvable process to one that is both preventable and, yes, reversible."

—DAVID PERLMUTTER, MD, AUTHOR OF THE #1 *New York Times* BESTSELLERS *Grain Brain* AND *Brain Maker*

"*The End of Alzheimer's* is a masterful, authoritative, and ultimately hopeful patient guide that will help you prevent and reverse Alzheimer's disease, whether you have the ApoE4 gene or not. My patients fear Alzheimer's more than any other diagnosis. This is the book to transmute fear into action."

—SARA GOTTFRIED, MD, AUTHOR OF THE *New York Times* BESTSELLER *Younger*

"Dr. Dale Bredesen is a world-class neuroscientist-neurologist who through his innovative and exacting research has discovered a safe and effective approach to the prevention and treatment of Alzheimer's disease that will revolutionize the way we think about the disease."

—JEFFREY BLAND, PhD, FOUNDER OF THE INSTITUTE FOR FUNCTIONAL MEDICINE, THE CLEVELAND CLINIC

"Dr. Bredesen has provided enormous hope for the heretofore intractable clinical problem of Alzheimer's. Bredesen's early studies suggest that this approach can halt and in many cases reverse early Alzheimer's."

—LEROY HOOD, MD, PhD, AWARDED THE NATIONAL MEDAL OF SCIENCE, PRESENTED BY PRESIDENT BARACK OBAMA IN 2011, AND FOUNDER OF THE INSTITUTE FOR SYSTEMS BIOLOGY

"Every citizen and medical professional interested in the brain and its health should read this seminal book. It should provide much of the basis for a true revolution in brain health medicine."

—MICHAEL MERZENICH, PhD, WINNER OF THE 2016 KAVLI PRIZE IN NEUROSCIENCE

"A must-read for anyone wondering what can be done for this dread disease, whether for themselves, a loved one, or a patient."

—NATHAN PRICE, PhD, PROFESSOR AND ASSOCIATE DIRECTOR OF THE INSTITUTE FOR SYSTEMS BIOLOGY

"Having spent several years implementing many of Dr. Bredesen's insights in my patients, I can assure you that following his advice can save yourself, your loved ones, and your friends from suffering from this preventable and reversible curse."

—STEVEN GUNDRY, MD, MEDICAL DIRECTOR OF THE INTERNATIONAL HEART AND LUNG INSTITUTE AND AUTHOR OF THE *New York Times* BESTSELLER *The Plant Paradox*

"This book represents a major turning point in our approach to Alzheimer's disease. For the first time ever, patients and families affected by Alzheimer's—as well as those at high risk for this devastating disease—truly have a reason to be hopeful."

—CHRIS KRESSER, MS, LAc, AUTHOR OF THE *New York Times* BESTSELLER *The Paleo Cure*

"*The End of Alzheimer's* offers a new beginning in medicine. Dr. Bredesen translates the knowledge of science to the wisdom that helps to heal our people . . . and provide a vision for the end of Alzheimer's."

—PATRICK HANAWAY, MD, FOUNDING MEDICAL DIRECTOR AND DIRECTOR OF RESEARCH, THE CENTER FOR FUNCTIONAL MEDICINE, THE CLEVELAND CLINIC

"An experimental program that some patients say has literally reversed their symptoms and allowed them to live a normal life."

—MARIA SHRIVER, APPEARING ON THE *Today* SHOW

"*The End of Alzheimer's*, for the first time, synthesizes the latest science into a practical plan that can reverse Alzheimer's and dramatically improve brain health and function. If you have a brain, read this book."

—MARK HYMAN, MD, DIRECTOR OF THE CENTER FOR FUNCTIONAL MEDICINE, THE CLEVELAND CLINIC, AND AUTHOR OF THE #1 *New York Times* BESTSELLER *Eat Fat, Get Thin*

"*The End of Alzheimer's* is a phenomenal book. Dr. Dale Bredesen's research is some of the most exciting work that I have seen in years and tackles the most important health issue of our time. This helps us understand this complex and devastating condition but is also the roadmap to prevent it in the first place. It is a must-read book. By tackling arguably the most important disease of our age, Dr. Dale Bredesen is actually changing the way we look at all chronic disease. This is a masterpiece."

—RANGAN CHATTERJEE, MbChB, BSc (HONS), MRCP, MRCGP

The End of Alzheimer's

The End of Alzheimer's

The First Programme to Prevent and Reverse the Cognitive Decline of Dementia

Dr Dale Bredesen

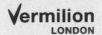

Vermilion
LONDON

3 5 7 9 10 8 6 4

Vermilion, an imprint of Ebury Publishing,

20 Vauxhall Bridge Road,

London SW1V 2SA

Vermilion is part of the Penguin Random House group of companies whose
addresses can be found at global.penguinrandomhouse.com

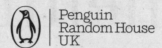

Penguin
Random House
UK

First published in the United Kingdom by Vermilion in 2017
First Published in the United States by Avery 2017

www.penguin.co.uk

A CIP catalogue record for this book is available from the British Library

ISBN 9781785041228

Printed and bound in India by Thomson Press India Ltd.

Penguin Random House is committed to a sustainable future for our business, our readers
and our planet. This book is made from Forest Stewardship Council® certified paper.

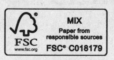

MIX
Paper from
responsible sources
FSC
www.fsc.org   FSC® C018179

This book is dedicated to my wife,
Dr. Aida Lasheen Bredesen—
a superb and caring physician who introduced me
to the world of functional and integrative medicine,
and who has taught me more than anyone
about this critical field—and to our two
beloved daughters, Tara and Tess.

Contents

PART FOUR

Maximizing Success

PART ONE

The Alzheimer's Solution

CHAPTER 1

Disrupting Dementia

*You never change things by fighting the existing reality.
To change something, build a new model that
makes the existing model obsolete.*
—R. BUCKMINSTER FULLER

IT IS IMPOSSIBLE to escape the drumbeat of grim news about Alzheimer's disease: that it is incurable and largely untreatable, that there is no reliable way to prevent it, and that the disease has for decades beaten the world's best neuroscientists. Despite the billions and billions of dollars spent by government agencies, pharmaceutical companies, and biotechnology wizards to invent and test drugs for Alzheimer's, 99.6 per cent of what we have come up with have been abysmal failures, not even making it out of the testing phase. And if you think there is hope in the 0.4 percent of discoveries that *have* reached the market—after all, we need only one Alzheimer's drug if it's effective, right?—think again. As the US Alzheimer's Association puts it in a bleak reality check, "A genuinely new Alzheimer's drug has not been approved since 2003, and the currently approved Alzheimer's medications are ineffective in stopping or slowing the course of the disease." Although the four available Alzheimer's drugs "may help lessen symptoms, such as memory loss and confusion," they do so only "for a limited time."

Maybe you're racking your memory to recall when you last read about the US Food and Drug Administration approving a new Alzheimer's drug. Don't worry if you can't: of 244 experimental Alzheimer's drugs tested from 2000 to 2010, exactly one— memantine—was approved, in 2003. And as I'll explain below, its effects are modest at best.

As I said, grim. No wonder a diagnosis of Alzheimer's disease is the last thing anyone wants to hear. One man whose wife was in the midst of the long goodbye of Alzheimer's shook his head, bereft, and said, "We are told repeatedly that drugs are being developed that will slow the decline—but why would anyone do that? I can tell you, living with this every day—that is the last thing you would want."

Alzheimer's disease has become part of the zeitgeist. In news articles and blogs and podcasts, on the radio and television and in films both documentary and fictional, we read and hear story after story about Alzheimer's disease. Sadly, all end tragically. We fear Alzheimer's as we fear no other disease. There are at least two reasons for that.

First, it is the only one—let me repeat that: *the only one*—of the Western world's ten most common causes of death for which there is no effective treatment. And by "effective," I am setting the bar pretty low. If we had a drug or other intervention that made people with Alzheimer's disease even a little better, never mind curing the disease, I'd sing its praises to the rooftops. So would everyone who has a loved one with Alzheimer's, everyone at risk for Alzheimer's, and of course everyone who has already developed Alzheimer's. But no such drug exists. We don't even have a treatment to keep people with subjective cognitive impairment or mild cognitive impairment (two conditions that often precede Alzheimer's disease) from going on to develop full-blown Alzheimer's.

Incredibly, given the astounding progress in other areas of medicine over the last twenty years—think cancer or HIV/AIDS or cystic fibrosis or cardiovascular disease—as I write this in 2017 not only is there no cure for Alzheimer's disease, there is not even anything that reliably prevents or slows Alzheimer's disease. You know how critics make fun of TV afternoon specials and Lifetime movies about angelic children or saintly mothers and fathers who bravely battled cancer and, with the aid of the latest miracle drug, are restored to perfect health before the final credits roll? Schmaltzy, sure. We in the Alzheimer's field would happily settle for schmaltzy if it were even remotely plausible to depict a happy ending to this disease.

The second reason Alzheimer's disease inspires such dread is because it's not "only" fatal. Lots of diseases are fatal. As the old joke has it, *life* is fatal. Alzheimer's is worse than fatal. For years and sometimes decades before it opens the door to the grim reaper, Alzheimer's disease robs its victims of their very humanity and terrorizes their families. Their memories, their capacity for thought, their ability to live full and independent lives—all gone, in a grim and unrelenting descent into a mental abyss where they no longer know their loved ones, their past, the world, or themselves.

The linguistics professor who is the heartbreaking protagonist of the 2014 movie *Still Alice* carries a DNA mutation that causes Alzheimer's disease to develop by middle age, discovered in 1995. You've probably read about the great strides that cancer biologists have made by discovering genes associated with tumors and crafting drugs based on them. With Alzheimer's disease? That 1995 discovery has not led to the development of a single Alzheimer's drug.

This awful disease stands out for one additional reason. The last fifty years have brought triumph after triumph in molecular biology and neuroscience. Biologists have untangled the immensely complex pathways that lead to cancer and have figured out how to block many of them. We have mapped out the chemical and electrical processes in the brain that underlie thoughts and feelings, developing effective, if imperfect, drugs for depression and schizophrenia, for anxiety and bipolar disorder. Sure, there's a lot left to be learned, and a lot of improvement needed for the compounds in our pharmacopoeias. But in virtually every other disease there is a strong sense that research is on the right track, that the basics are understood, that although nature will keep throwing curve balls at us, she has revealed to us the fundamental rules of the game. Not so with Alzheimer's.

In this disease, it's as if nature handed us a rule book written in disappearing ink and edited by evil gremlins who rewrite entire sections when our backs are turned. What I mean is this: seemingly rock-solid evidence from lab rodents suggested that Alzheimer's disease is caused by the accumulation in the brain of sticky synapse-destroying plaques made of a piece of a protein called amyloid-beta. Those lab studies indicated that amyloid-beta is formed in the brain by a series of steps, and that either intervening in those steps or destroying amyloid-beta* plaques would be an effective way to treat and even prevent Alzheimer's disease. Since the 1980s most neurobiologists have treated this basic idea, called the amyloid hypothesis, as dogma. It has won its developers multimillion-dollar prizes, countless accolades, and prestigious academic positions. It has had a huge influence on which Alzheimer's papers get published in top medical journals (hint: preference goes to those that toe the amyloid line) and

_____

* For simplicity, I'll henceforth refer to amyloid-beta as simply amyloid.

what studies get funded by the U.S. National Institutes of Health, the nation's chief source of support for biomedical research (ditto).

But here's the thing: when drug companies tested compounds that are based on any piece of the amyloid hypothesis, the results have ranged from frustrating to bewildering. In clinical trials, human brains did not respond to these compounds the way the rule book said they should. It would be one thing if the compounds failed to do what they were designed to do. That wasn't what happened. In many cases the compounds (usually, antibodies that bind to amyloid in an attempt to remove it) did a great job at removing amyloid plaques. Or if the compound was designed to block the enzyme needed to produce amyloid, it did a great job at that. The experimental compounds did precisely what their inventors intended, following the amyloid rule book, *but patients either got no better or, incredibly, got worse.* What keeps emerging from these clinical trials (which, by the way, often cost upward of £38 million each) is exactly the opposite of what all the test-tube research based on the amyloid hypothesis and all the mouse models of the amyloid hypothesis and all the theories of the amyloid hypothesis predicted. Targeting amyloid was supposed to be the golden ticket to curing Alzheimer's. It wasn't.

It's as if our space rockets exploded on the launchpad every single time.

Something is enormously wrong here.

Just as tragic as the blinkered adherence to the amyloid hypothesis is mainstream medicine's assumption that Alzheimer's is a *single* disease. As such, it is typically treated with *donepezil (Aricept Eisai/Pfizer)* and/or *memantine (Ebixa, Lundbeck).* I know I said that there is currently no treatment for Alzheimer's disease, so let me explain.

Donepezil (Aricept) is what's called a cholinesterase inhibitor*: it keeps a particular enzyme (cholinesterase) from destroying acetylcholine, a type of brain chemical called a neurotransmitter. Neurotransmitters carry signals from one neuron to another, which is how we think, remember, feel, and move, and so is important for memory and overall brain function. The rationale is simple: in Alzheimer's disease, there is a reduction in acetylcholine. Therefore, if you block the enzyme (cholinesterase) that breaks down acetylcholine, more will remain in your synapses. Then, even as Alzheimer's is ravaging the brain, the synapses might remain functional a little while longer.

To a modest extent, this rationale does work, but there are important caveats. First, blocking the breakdown of acetylcholine does not affect the cause or progression of Alzheimer's disease. The disease therefore still progresses. Second, the brain often responds to inhibition of cholinesterase as you might expect: by making more cholinesterase. That obviously limits the drugs' efficacy (and can become a real problem if the drug is stopped suddenly). Third, like all drugs, cholinesterase inhibitors have side effects; they include diarrhoea, nausea and vomiting, headache, joint pain, drowsiness, loss of appetite, and bradycardia (slowed heart rate).

As for memantine, it too acts on brain chemicals and molecules that have little to do with fundamental Alzheimer's pathophysiology, but, like Aricept, might reduce (or even delay) the symptoms of the disease, at least for a time. It is typically used later in the disease, but may be used in combination with a cholinesterase inhibitor. Memantine inhibits the transmission of brain signals from one neuron to the next via the neurotransmitter glutamate. Inhibiting that transmission reduces what's called

---

* Other cholinesterase inhibitors prescribed for Alzheimer's disease include rivastigmine (Exelon), galantamine (Reminyl), and huperzine A (available online).

glutamate's excitotoxic effect, meaning the toxic effect associated with neuronal activation. Unfortunately, memantine may also inhibit the very neurotransmission critical to memory formation, and so may initially impair cognitive function.

Most important, neither cholinesterase inhibitors nor memantine gets at the underlying causes of Alzheimer's or stops the disease from worsening—and they certainly do not cure it.

All of that is bad enough, but there is a more fundamental problem. Alzheimer's is *not* a single disease. Sure, the symptoms might make it look like it is, but as I explain in chapter 6, we discovered that there are three main subtypes of Alzheimer's. Our research on the different biochemical profiles of people with Alzheimer's has made it clear that these three readily distinguishable subtypes are each driven by different biochemical processes. Each one requires a different treatment. Treating them all the same way is as naive as treating every infection with the same antibiotic.

It's bad enough that Alzheimer's disease has, for more than thirty years, defeated the greatest minds in neuroscience and medicine. (I'm not counting the seventy-plus years between when the disease was named and when the amyloid hypothesis emerged; much less research was done on Alzheimer's disease in those decades.) Anyone who pays attention can see that we're using the wrong approach. In particular, the idea of identifying the *cause* of the amyloid production, removing that, and then removing the amyloid, has not been tested.

If you have a high risk of developing Alzheimer's because of the genes you carry, if you have already developed it, or if you have a loved one who has, you therefore have every right to be very upset about this situation.

No wonder we have come to fear Alzheimer's disease as omnipotent. As hopeless. As impervious to any and all treatments.

Until now.

Let me say this as clearly as I can: *Alzheimer's disease can be prevented, and in many cases its associated cognitive decline can be reversed.* For that is precisely what my colleagues and I have shown in peer-reviewed studies in leading medical journals—studies that, for the first time, describe exactly this remarkable result in patients. Yes, I know it flouts decades of conventional wisdom to claim that cognitive decline can be reversed, that there are hundreds of patients who have done just that, and that there are steps we can all take now to prevent the cognitive decline that experts have long believed to be unavoidable and irreversible. These are bold claims deserving of healthy scepticism. I expect you to exercise that scepticism as you read about the three decades of research in my lab, which culminated in the first reversals of cognitive decline in early Alzheimer's disease and its precursors, MCI (mild cognitive impairment) and SCI (subjective cognitive impairment). I expect you to exercise that scepticism as you read the stories of these patients, patients who climbed out of the abyss of cognitive decline. I expect you to exercise that scepticism as you read about the personalized therapeutic programmes we developed to enable everyone to prevent cognitive impairment and, if they are already showing signs of it, to stop mental decline in its tracks and restore their ability to remember, to think, and to once again live a cognitively healthy life.

But if the results I describe overcome your scepticism, then please open your mind and consider changing your life—not only if you have already begun the slide into cognitive decline, but even if you haven't. Needless to say, the people who will find this book most immediately and directly life-changing are those whose memory and cognition are already suffering (and their family members and caretakers). By following the protocol I describe, those with cognitive impairment that is not yet Alzheimer's disease, as well as those who are already in the grip of Alzheimer's, can not only halt but often actually reverse the cognitive decline they have already suffered. For those so stricken, progression to severe dementia has until now been inevitable, with nothing but bad news from every expert. The anti-Alzheimer's protocol my colleagues and I developed consigns that bleak dogma to the dustbin of history.

There is a second, very specific group for whom this book can mean the difference between the grim future they have probably been told to expect and a future filled with health and joy. These are the people who carry a gene variant (allele) called ApoE4 (ApoE is short for apolipoprotein E; an apolipoprotein is a protein that carries lipids—i.e., fats). ApoE4 is the strongest known genetic risk factor* for Alzheimer's disease. Carrying one ApoE4 (that is, inherited from one parent) increases your lifetime risk of Alzheimer's to 30 per cent, while carrying two copies (inheriting copies from both parents) increases it to well over 50 per cent (from 50 to 90 per cent, depending on which study you read). That compares to a risk of only about 9 per cent in people who carry zero copies of this allele.

The vast majority of ApoE4 carriers don't know about this potential ticking time bomb in their DNA, and typically find out only after the onset of symptoms of Alzheimer's disease spur them to undergo genetic testing. It is certainly understandable that, as long as there is no prevention or treatment for Alzheimer's, most people would not want to know their ApoE status. In fact, when Nobel laureate Dr. James Watson (codiscoverer of the DNA double helix) had his genome sequenced in 2007, he said he did not wish to be told whether he carried ApoE4; why expose yourself to devastating news if there's nothing you can do about it? However, now that there is a programme that can

---

* Other genes, called presenilin-1 (PS1) and presenilin-2 (PS2), also increase the risk of Alzheimer's, and almost always cause symptoms to develop before age 60 and as early as a person's thirties. But these genes have been found in only a few hundred extended families, accounting for less than 5 per cent of cases.

reduce the risk of Alzheimer's, even in those carrying ApoE4, dramatic reductions in the prevalence of dementia could be achieved if more people underwent genetic testing to determine their ApoE status and initiated a preventive programme long before any symptoms appeared. It is my fervent hope that this is exactly what will happen, and that ApoE4 carriers in particular learn from this book that their situation is not hopeless: you too can take steps to prevent Alzheimer's disease or reverse cognitive decline.

There is a perhaps less obvious group, for whom I believe this book can be life-changing: everyone past the age of 40. The number one concern of individuals as we age (and yes, when we talk about brain aging, the downhill slide begins at about 40) is the loss of our cognitive abilities. For it is those abilities—to read a letter from a loved one and comprehend it; to watch a movie or read a book and follow the plot; to observe the people in our lives and understand them; to perceive the events around us and maintain a sense of our place in the world; to perform the basic functions of daily life so we are not mere sacks of protoplasm dependent on others to feed, dress, move, and bathe us; to remember the events of our life and the people who have been precious to it— that define us as human. When they go, so does our very identity as someone with a meaningful life. To all of you lucky enough to have avoided even a hint of these losses even as you are acutely aware that they may be lurking in your future, my message is this: take a deep breath and realize that cognitive decline is—at least for most of us and, especially, early in its course—addressable. Despite what you may have been told, it is not hopeless or irreversible. To the contrary. For the first time, hope and Alzheimer's have come together.

And the reason for that is one fundamental discovery: Alzheimer's "disease" is not the result of the brain doing something it isn't supposed to do, the way cancer is the result of cells proliferating out of control or heart disease is the result of blood vessels getting clogged with atherosclerotic plaque. Alzheimer's arises from an intrinsic and healthy downsizing programme for your brain's extensive synaptic network. But it is a programme that has run amok, sort of the way Mickey Mouse's efforts to get enchanted brooms to carry buckets of water for him in "The Sorcerer's Apprentice" segment of the 1940 classic *Fantasia* eventually lead to the brooms running amok. In Alzheimer's, an otherwise normal brain-housekeeping process has gone haywire.

THIS BOOK IS not a scientific tome—though I include the scientific evidence that supports my conclusions—but instead a practical, easy-to-use, step-by-step manual for preventing and reversing the cognitive decline of early Alzheimer's disease or its precursors, mild cognitive impairment and subjective cognitive impairment, and for sustaining that improvement. It is also a guidebook by which the many millions who carry the ApoE4 gene can escape the fate written in their DNA. The protocol for achieving this led to the first-ever scientific publication of a study, in 2014,* reporting the reversal of cognitive decline in patients nine out of ten of them—with Alzheimer's disease or its precursors, thanks to a sophisticated personalized protocol based on our decades of research on the neurobiology of Alzheimer's disease. Called ReCODE,† for reversal of cognitive decline, the protocol not only achieved the reversal of cognitive decline in Alzheimer's disease and pre-Alzheimer's that no one thought possible; it also allowed patients to sustain that improvement. The very first patient treated with what is now the ReCODE protocol is, as I write

---

* Three subsequent scientific papers, in 2015 and 2016, have confirmed that first study.
† The method was initially called MEND, for metabolic enhancement for neurodegeneration. But MEND is now out-of-date, having been replaced by our more advanced ReCODE protocol.

this, five years into the treatment, and at 73 remains cognitively healthy, travelling the world and working full-time. Our extensive subsequent work, with hundreds of patients, proves that she is far from unique.

After publication of the 2014 study, we received many thousands of emails, phone calls, and visits from physicians and other practitioners, potential patients, and family members from all over the United States, the UK, Australia, Asia, Europe, and South America, wanting to learn more about the successful protocol. The journal that had published the study is called *Aging*, and the staff called to inform us that, of the tens of thousands of scientific papers the journal had published over the years, ours had scored in the top couple—and thus in the 99.99th percentile—in the system of metrics that gauges impact and interest. Although in that initial scientific paper I did not include a detailed step-by-step description of the protocol (scientific journals have page limitations for each paper), in this book I do. I also recount how I developed ReCODE and explain its scientific basis. In the appendix, I list sources of the foods, supplements, and other components of ReCODE as well as links to doctors and other healthcare practitioners who are knowledgeable about it and can help you implement it in your own life—or in the life of a loved one.

There is nothing more important than making a difference in the lives of patients, and that is what has driven me in the decades-long quest to find a way to prevent and reverse Alzheimer's disease. But if enough people adopt ReCODE, they will be helping far more than themselves. Because Alzheimer's disease strikes an estimated one in nine Americans 65 and older, or 5.2 million people as I write this, the aging of the baby boom generation threatens to bring a tsunami of Alzheimer's immense enough to bankrupt Medicare and Medicaid and overwhelm the US's long-term care facilities—to say nothing of the toll it will take on tens of millions of families whose loved ones are swallowed by this merciless disease. (It will also be catastrophic for the NHS in the UK.) Globally, a projected 160 million people will, by 2050, develop Alzheimer's. That makes the need for prevention and treatment greater than ever. The hundreds of patients I have seen battle back from cognitive decline—battle back despite the medical dogma that such a recovery is impossible—have convinced me that the prevention and treatment of Alzheimer's is not some pie-in-the-sky fantasy.

We know how to do it—now, today.

That's what I mean when I say that if enough people adopt ReCODE, the consequences would ripple across the nation and the world, cutting medical costs by many billions of pounds a year, preventing a crisis in the NHS, reducing the global burden of dementia, and enhancing longevity. All of these are feasible.

Here, finally, is nothing less than the first good news about Alzheimer's disease. It is a chronicle of joy, of the blessing of getting your life back. One of the patients you shall read about said he has allowed himself to think about the future once again when he talks to his grandchildren. Another said her memory is better than it has been in thirty years. One musician's wife said his guitar playing has returned; the daughter of another said her mother, who had been disappearing slowly each time the daughter returned from college, is once again part of the family. What you read about here is the beginning of a changed world, the beginning of the end of Alzheimer's disease.

Here's what's ahead:

Chapters 2 to 6 relate the scientific odyssey that led to ReCODE. They describe the discoveries that form the scientific basis of the treatment protocol—what Alzheimer's disease actually looks like "under the hood," where it comes from, and why it is so common. These are the discoveries that support the first effective approach to preventing cognitive decline, identifying the metabolic and other factors that increase your risk, and reversing cognitive decline if it has already begun. These are also the discoveries that challenge the central dogma of Alzheimer's: they showed that this devastating disease is the result of a normal, healthy brain process that has gone haywire. That is, the brain suffers some injury, infection, or other assault (I'll explain the many kinds) and responds by defending itself. The defence mechanism includes producing the Alzheimer's-associated amyloid. Yes, you read that correctly—the amyloid that has been vilified for decades, the very amyloid that everyone has been trying to get rid of, is part of a *protective* response. No wonder trying to get rid of it hasn't been very helpful to those with Alzheimer's disease.

Contrary to the current dogma, therefore, what is referred to as Alzheimer's disease is actually a protective response to, specifically, three different processes: inflammation, suboptimal levels of nutrients and other synapse-supporting molecules, and toxic exposures. I'll say more about each of these in chapter 6, but for now, let me underline this simple message: the realization that Alzheimer's disease can exist in three distinct subtypes (and often in combinations of these subtypes) has profound implications for the way we evaluate, prevent, and treat it. That discovery also means that we can better treat the subtler forms of cognitive loss, mild cognitive impairment and subjective cognitive impairment, before they progress to full-blown Alzheimer's disease.

In chapter 7, you'll learn about the tests that identify what is causing your cognitive decline or putting you at risk for it—how you may already be giving yourself Alzheimer's disease. The tests are necessary because the often numerous contributors to one person's cognitive decline are very likely different from the contributors to someone else's. These tests therefore give you a personalized risk profile, letting you know which factors to address to optimize improvement. You will learn the rationale behind each test—that is, how the physiological parameter it evaluates contributes to brain function and Alzheimer's disease. Chapter 7 summarizes the tests involved in this "cognoscopy" and explains the guiding principles behind them.

Chapters 8 and 9 explain what to do in response to the test results. These discuss the fundamentals that must be addressed in order to reverse cognitive decline and reduce risk for future decline: inflammation/infection, insulin resistance, hormone and supportive nutrient depletion, toxin exposure, and the replacement and protection of lost or dysfunctional brain connections (synapses). This is not a "one size fits all" approach. Everyone's version of Re-CODE is personalized, based on their test results: your version will be different from that of others because it is optimized to your unique physiology. Of course, the very fact that ReCODE works—that it prevents and reverses cognitive decline—makes it unique and novel. But so does its focus on personalization.

In chapters 10 through 12, I explain the keys to achieving the very best results and to sustaining that improvement. These chapters offer workarounds, not only to help you succeed in reversing cognitive decline, but also to address the questions and criticism that have been directed at this approach.

Since the advent of "modern" medicine in the nineteenth century, doctors have been trained to diagnose disease—for example, hypertension or congestive heart failure or arthritis—and prescribe a standard one-size-fits-all treatment, such as an antihypertensive for hypertension. That is slowly changing, as with precision cancer treatments in which the genetic profile of a patient's tumour dictates what drug to prescribe. The push for personalized medicine could bring us closer to a core aspect of Eastern medicine such as TCM (traditional Chinese medicine) and Ayurvedic medicine: although the ancient practitioners of these healing traditions were not aware of the molecular biological details of particular diseases, they were experts at treating the whole person instead of focusing on a single "disease" such as hypertension.

The new medicine—twenty-first-century medicine—brings together the best of the modern Western and the traditional Eastern approaches. It combines a knowledge of molecular mechanisms with an understanding of the entire person. This allows us to go beyond simply asking *what* the problem is to asking *why* the problem is. Asking *why* makes all the difference—including, as you'll see, in the prevention and treatment of Alzheimer's disease.

What the research from my laboratory colleagues and me adds up to is this: No one should die from Alzheimer's disease. Let me say that again: *No one should die from Alzheimer's disease.* To accomplish this will require that we—clinicians as well as patients—update our practices from twentieth-century medicine to twenty-first-century medicine, and that we be proactive about our own cognitive and general health.

Books on medical science are supposed to be dispassionate, objective expositions of "facts," as peer-reviewed and approved by the experts, so I beg your indulgence for failing to remain completely dispassionate. As history has proven time and again, all too often the facts that we as a biomedical and scientific community accept, endorse, and propagate as gospel turn out ultimately to be incorrect. (Newborns cannot feel pain. Ulcers are caused by stress. Hormone replacement therapy for postmenopausal women prevents heart disease. And on and on.) The field of neurodegenerative diseases has not been immune from such recursive crashing and burning of its own dogmatic assertions. Depending on which expert you ask and when, Alzheimer's disease is due to free radicals or metal binding or misfolded proteins or diabetes of the brain or tau protein or detergent-like effects or . . . well, the list goes on. There is simply no consensus. Moreover, none of the current hypotheses explains all of the published data, which is contained in more than 50,000 published papers. Is it any wonder that Alzheimer's disease is on track to take the lives of 45 million of the 325 million Americans alive today?

So yes, I am very passionate about this cause, this disease, the underlying neurodegenerative process, the many overly simplistic approaches taken to address it, the political and financial nature of the decisions made, and the millions dying. As doctors, we worry that sentiment and passion may colour our medical decisions, robbing us of objectivity. This is an appropriate concern. However, anyone following the Alzheimer's field, watching the heartbreak and desperation, might rationally conclude that *dis*passion colours far too many of our daily decisions. Have we as a society become numb to the tragedy of dementia? Have we given up on trying to pull out all the stops? Have we decided that the same kind of scientific genius that developed cardiac bypass, antibiotics, plasmapheresis, artificial limbs, stem cells, and organ transplants is powerless against Alzheimer's disease? Are we, as scientists and clinicians, such prisoners of medical dogma that we focus completely on single-drug, one-size-fits-all approaches to Alzheimer's no matter how many times they fail?

I hope not, for if necessity is indeed the mother of invention, then perhaps passion is its father.

CHAPTER 2

Patient Zero

*"Everyone knows a cancer survivor; no one
knows an Alzheimer's survivor."*

MEET KRISTIN.

Kristin was suicidal. Years before, she had watched in despair as her mother's mind slipped away, forcing her to enter a nursing home after she could no longer recognize family members, let alone care for herself. Kristin had suffered along with her mother, who at the age of 62 had begun an 18-year decline into Alzheimer's disease. And at the end Kristin had suffered alone, for her mother was no longer sentient.

When Kristin was 65, she began to experience her own cognitive problems. She got lost when driving on the freeway, unable to remember where to get off and on, even on familiar routes. She could no longer analyze data critical to her job, or organize and prepare reports in a timely fashion. Unable to remember numbers, she had to write down even four digits, not to mention phone numbers. She had trouble remembering what she had read, and by the time she reached the bottom of a page had to start at the top again. Reluctantly, Kristin prepared her resignation. She began to make mistakes more and more frequently, often calling her pets by the wrong names and having to search to find the light switches in her own home, even though she had flipped them on and off for years.

Like many people, Kristin tried to ignore these symptoms. But they got worse and worse. After two years of unremitting cognitive decline, she consulted her doctor, who told her she was becoming demented just as her mother had, and there was nothing he could do for her. He wrote "memory problems" on her chart, and because of that, she was unable to obtain long-term care insurance. She underwent retinal scanning, which revealed the Alzheimer's-associated amyloid. She thought about the horror of watching her mother decline, about how she would live with progressive dementia and no long-term care, about the lack of treatment. She decided to commit suicide.

She called her best friend, Barbara, explaining, "I watched what my mother went through as she slipped away, and there is no way I will allow that to happen to me." Barbara was horrified to hear Kristin's saga. But unlike when other friends had fallen victim to dementia, this time Barbara had an idea. She told Kristin about new research she had heard about, and suggested that rather than ending her life, Kristin travel several thousand miles to the Buck Institute for Research on Aging, just north of San Francisco. In 2012, Kristin came to see me.

We talked for hours. I could offer her no guarantee, no example of any patient who had used the protocol— nothing more than diagrams, theory, and data from transgenic mice. In reality, Barbara had been premature in sending her to the Institute. And to make matters worse, the protocol I had developed had just been turned down for its first proposed clinical trial. The review board felt that it was "too complicated," and pointed out that such trials are meant to test only a single drug or intervention, not an entire programme (ah, if only diseases were that simple!). So all I could do was to go over the various parts of the protocol and recommend that she take these to her doctor back home, asking him if he would work with her. She did that, and so began what has become the ReCODE protocol.

Three months later, Kristin called me at home on a Saturday to say she could not believe the changes in her mental abilities. She was able to work full-time again, to drive without getting lost, and to remember phone numbers without difficulty. She was feeling better than she had in years. When I put the phone down, what rushed into my mind were the decades of research, the countless hours at the whiteboard with lab members and colleagues, the arguments with myself about each detail of the theory and treatment approach. All of this had not been in vain; it had pointed us in the right direction. Of course Kristin was only one person—as they say, an "n of one"—and we needed to see similar results in thousands and ultimately in millions. I thought back to the doctor who told his patient, "You are just an anecdote; you are not statistically significant." To which his patient replied, "Well, my family says that I *am* significant. Besides, I'm healthy once again, so I don't care about statistics." Indeed. Every fundamental change needs to start somewhere—every successful approach must start with Patient Zero—and Kristin was Patient Zero.

She confided in a family member, "Did you know I had Alzheimer's disease?" He said, "Of course, it was obvious. I just did not want to say anything to you about it—I did not want to make you feel bad." Kristin, who is now 73, has been on ReCODE for five years. She still works full-time, travels the world, and continues to be asymptomatic. Furthermore, she has discontinued the programme, albeit briefly, four times, for various reasons—a brief viral illness, running out of some of the pills, travelling—and each time her cognition began to decline. But when she resumed ReCODE, it again returned to normal.

When my colleagues and I started the research that led to ReCODE in 1989, the Alzheimer's dogma was well established. The disease, according to the theory that has prevailed since the 1980s, is caused by sticky gobs or plaques of amyloid, a protein molecule, gunking up the spaces between brain neurons. Since these spaces, or synapses, are where neurons communicate with one another, the damage caused by the sticky amyloid plaques has devastating consequences: synapses stop functioning. Indeed, the amyloid plaques were one of the abnormalities that neuropathologist Dr. Aloysius Alzheimer (1864–1915) saw in the autopsied brain of the first patient he diagnosed with presenile dementia, as he described it in 1906. (The other abnormality was a profusion of long stringy tangles of proteins called tau, but the importance of these neurofibrillary tangles has long been over-shadowed by the focus on amyloid plaques.) The dominance of the amyloid hypothesis led to a herd mentality. Many experimental compounds developed to treat Alzheimer's worked the same way, by grabbing hold of the amyloid plaques (or in some cases of amyloid before it had stuck together into plaques) and attempting to remove it.

Scientists at medical centres, universities, and pharmaceutical and biotechnology companies have discovered hundreds of these amyloid-removing compounds. Scores of them looked promising enough in laboratory animals that powerhouse pharmaceutical companies such as Eli Lilly and Biogen have spent billions of dollars to test them in patients, in clinical trials. I don't have to hedge or estimate when I tell you how many of the 200-plus experimental drugs have proven safe and effective enough in these trials—where *effective* means they have stopped the worsening of or, even better, reversed Alzheimer's disease—to be approved by the US Food and Drug Administration. That number is zero. Hence, according to the US Alzheimer's Association, no drug "can cure Alzheimer's or stop it from progressing."

Of course, all of these failures have cast doubt on what has been the central dogma in Alzheimer's research, which is called the amyloid cascade hypothesis. This suggests that amyloid plays a central role in Alzheimer's disease, which is a bit like saying that lumps of cells play a central role in cancer—it doesn't tell you why the amyloid is there, what its normal function is, or how to prevent the disease. Most important, it doesn't tell you what Alzheimer's disease actually *is*.

Not surprisingly, while early results in Kristin and a handful of other patients on ReCODE led to a stampede of requests for more information from doctors, patients, and patients' families, they also led to intense scepticism. That's because they flew in the face of the long held dogma that nothing will prevent, slow, or reverse Alzheimer's disease—at least not until the first miracle drug arrives, and certainly not something like ReCODE's extensive protocol. But the number of patients successfully treated with Re-CODE is now over 200, and more and more medical professionals are using it successfully for their own patients. Since 2016 I have trained some 450 doctors, neuropsychologists, nurses, health coaches, and nutritional therapists from 7 different countries and throughout the United States in this approach.

Even more encouraging, increasing numbers of neuroscientists and doctors are beginning to recognize that Alzheimer's disease is not what we thought it was. Rather than being caused by the buildup of those sticky amyloid plaques (or neuron-strangling tangles), the disease we call Alzheimer's is actually the result of a *protective response* in the brain.

This is worth repeating. *Alzheimer's disease does not arise from the brain failing to function as it evolved to.* It is not like cancer, where a genetic mutation—inherited or acquired during the course of life—turns a cell and all its progeny into out-of-control proliferators that take over an organ. It is not like rheumatoid arthritis and other autoimmune diseases, where the immune system turns on the body's own cells and attacks them. In those and many other diseases, something is dangerously out of whack: a physiological system is not functioning as intended.

Alzheimer's is different. As I explain in detail in chapter 4, one of the key discoveries to come out of my lab is that Alzheimer's arises when the brain *responds as it should* to certain threats. Why would evolution give us a brain that works like this? Because in most cases this response to outside threats succeeds; the brain beats back the threat and goes on functioning just fine. The problem comes when those threats are chronic, multiple, unrelenting, and intense. In this situation, the defences that the brain mounts are also chronic, multiple, unrelenting, and intense—so much so that these protective mechanisms cross the line into causing harm. Specifically, Alzheimer's disease is what happens when the brain tries to protect itself from three metabolic and toxic threats:

- Inflammation (from infection, diet, or other causes)
- Decline and shortage of supportive nutrients, hormones, and other brain-supporting molecules
- Toxic substances such as metals or biotoxins (poisons produced by microbes such as moulds)

In chapter 6 I will explain in detail how we discovered that these three types of threats—which have dozens of contributors— trigger this protective response in the brain—including what the three kinds of threats do and why the amyloid response that they incite is so toxic to the brain's synapses. But for now let me simply say that once we recognize that Alzheimer's disease is what happens when the brain struggles to defend itself against inflammation, to function despite a shortage of beneficial compounds, or to fight an influx of toxic substances, the optimal way to prevent and treat the disease becomes clear: identify which of the many potential contributors to these three classes of threats a particular patient's brain is responding to defensively, remove the specific contributors, and help it fend off the remaining attackers.

That means that in order to reverse cognitive decline in subjective cognitive impairment, mild cognitive impairment, or Alzheimer's disease (and potentially in other forms of dementia such as Lewy body disease), it is necessary to remove the factors— preferably all of them in each of the three categories—that are causing our brains to defend themselves by producing the protective amyloid response. After removing the three kinds of threats, the next step is to remove the amyloid itself. Once you've eliminated the triggers for amyloid production plus the amyloid that has already been produced, you need to rebuild the synapses that the disease has destroyed.

If all of this makes you think there is not a one-size-fits-all regimen for treating subjective cognitive impairment, mild cognitive impairment, and Alzheimer's disease, you're right. However, since we're all vulnerable to each of the triggers and have no way of knowing which one (or two or all three) might assault our brain, it's important to reduce your chances of all of them—of inflammation, of a shortage of supportive compounds, and of exposure to neurotoxic substances. If you already have SCI, MCI, or Alzheimer's disease, it's crucial to determine which of the readily distinguishable subtypes—caused by inflammation, by a dearth of brain-supporting molecules, or by toxic compounds— you have, since each subtype has its own optimal treatment, and in fact each person's profile dictates a personalized optimal treatment.

For this reason the effective prevention and reversal of cognitive decline in Alzheimer's disease involves the new field of programmatics, which means that developing optimal treatments for complex chronic illnesses such as Alzheimer's disease involves identifying the many contributors for each person and then fashioning the best programme to target these contributors. The reason we have to enlist programmatics to fight Alzheimer's is simple: the many contributors to cognitive decline render the single-pill approach—monotherapeutics—marginally helpful at best, and usually ineffective.

Let me emphasize that your brain health is largely affected by these three kinds of disturbances and your ability to thwart them in the first place or drive them off if they have already taken hold in your brain. Fortunately, there are relatively easy ways to identify, measure, and treat each of the three disturbances in order to optimize brain function.

Our bodies are complex systems. Rather than viewing the brain as an organ distinct from the rest of the body, we must recognize that our cells and physiological systems work as a whole. What makes one system flourish or fail often makes other, seemingly unrelated systems also flourish or fail. By preventing and, if necessary, righting imbalances in our basic biochemistry, we can prevent and improve dysfunctions *before* a disease has taken over. Targeting a symptom that appears after a disease has taken hold, as most conventional methods do, is very different from attacking the root cause of a disease at the cellular level. In other words, we want to get to the cause of cognitive decline, fixing any imbalances before it becomes irreversible.

Fair warning: Treating your whole system is necessarily more complex than treating a symptom or single problem. There are many potential factors or abnormalities that contribute to cognitive decline, or even to the risk of cognitive decline. We initially identified thirty-six, and have since identified a few more, but results to date suggest that there are not many more—certainly not thousands or even hundreds. Effective prevention and early

Terminology

Dementia: A global cognitive decline in which many mental abilities are lost. Memory loss is often one of the earlier symptoms, which typically include difficulty with reading, writing, speaking, following a conversation, reasoning, calculating, organizing, and planning. There are many causes of dementia, including vascular dementia, frontotemporal dementia, Lewy body dementia, and others, but Alzheimer's disease is the most common. ReCODE has been shown to help with Alzheimer's disease and pre-Alzheimer's disease (SCI and MCI, described below), but we do not yet know whether it may be helpful with other causes of dementia, such as Lewy body disease.

Vascular dementia: The form of dementia caused by reduced blood flow to the brain and marked by multiple small strokes. In recent years it has been recognized that Alzheimer's disease and vascular dementia overlap somewhat.

Frontotemporal dementia: This is much less common than Alzheimer's disease, and often features changes in behaviour, memory problems, and difficulty speaking.

Lewy body dementia: This is a fairly common cause of dementia (about one patient for every five Alzheimer's patients), and features visual hallucinations, delusions, increased sleeping, and flinging of limbs during sleep (called REM behavioral disturbance), among other features.

Alzheimer's disease: This form of dementia is marked by amyloid plaques and neurofibrillary tangles. As explained in the text, there is growing evidence that neither is the cause of Alzheimer's, as long believed, but nevertheless Alzheimer's disease is typically diagnosed by looking for plaques and tangles. Neither can be seen directly in the living brain, but forms of neuroimaging such as PET (positron-emission tomography), as well as analysis of cerebrospinal fluid, can identify their presence. Alzheimer's disease is usually diagnosed on the basis of a patient's symptoms, which include memory loss and cognitive deficits so severe and ever-worsening that the patient loses the ability to bathe, eat, or dress without assistance and is increasingly unable to care for himself or herself. With the current standard treatment, Alzheimer's is invariably fatal.

Subjective cognitive impairment (SCI): Worsening cognition that is noticeable to the individual but, in standard neuropsychological testing, still falls in the normal range. A very intelligent individual may recognize his or her memory loss only to be told that testing shows his or her memory to be in the "normal" range, but this "normal" actually represents a decline from the person's earlier ability. Even at this early stage, PET scans and cerebrospinal fluid will often be abnormal, and MRI (magnetic resonance imaging) may show some shrinkage of brain regions. SCI often lasts a decade or so before progressing to MCI.

Mild cognitive impairment (MCI): This typically follows subjective cognitive impairment. Neuropsychological tests show that memory, organizing, speaking, calculating, planning, or other cognitive abilities are abnormal, but the person is still able to perform the so-called activities of daily living, such as dressing, eating, and bathing. MCI does not inevitably progress to Alzheimer's disease, but in many people, especially those in whom memory loss is part of their MCI, Alzheimer's disease will follow within a few years.

reversal requires knowing the status of each factor—if you have been exposed to specific toxins in mould called mycotoxins, for instance, or if the concentration of inflammatory molecules in your blood is too high. The ReCODE protocol provides a way to assess these factors and, based on that, provides an individualized treatment plan.

CHAPTER 3

How Does It Feel to Come Back from Dementia?

War would end if the dead could return.
—STANLEY BALDWIN

W E ALL LEARN as children that when you're sick, you feel bad. That's what keeps you out of school and why you go to the doctor: you feel lousy. Feeling lousy and illness go hand in hand, right? That's the problem with Alzheimer's disease. You go for a long, long time *without* feeling lousy, so by the time you have symptoms noticeable enough to send you to a doctor, the disease is relatively far along and difficult, if not impossible, to treat. With Alzheimer's, the underlying disease process is typically ongoing for fifteen to twenty years before a diagnosis is made.

To make matters worse, when we do develop symptoms such as memory loss, we tend to look for excuses to assure ourselves that nothing serious is going on. We talk about words being "on the tip of the tongue" or about having a "senior moment." We say we'll "think of it in a minute," are having a momentary "brain cramp," or are taking an "intellectual pause." In fairness, many of us who have such momentary lapses are not suffering from early Alzheimer's disease and so should not be unduly concerned. However, others of us are.

If you could come *back* from Alzheimer's disease, what would you report about the feeling of descent into dementia? And on a more positive note, how would it feel to get your abilities back? Thanks to the many people who have returned to normal on the ReCODE protocol, we can finally get answers to these questions and others. This is not to say that each person has the same early symptoms, nor that each patient's recovery follows the same trajectory. However, each person's experience has something to teach us.

Eleanor, for instance, was only 40 years old when she began getting pulled into the black hole of Alzheimer's disease. Her father was in the late stages of Alzheimer's disease when Eleanor started to notice in herself the same symptoms he had developed years earlier:

1. *Facial blindness.* Difficulty recognizing and remembering faces, called prosopagnosia, was the first change Eleanor noticed, and it seemed to come on suddenly and noticeably around the time she turned 40. "I didn't connect this to early dementia," she told me, "but to fatigue or a sort of learning disability (though I don't remember having this problem when I was younger). My dad had this as well."

2. *Decreasing mental clarity (especially later in the day).* "I started to experience a growing mental 'fatigue,' especially after three or four P.M. I mistakenly thought I was just very tired. Helping my kids with homework felt mentally exhausting. It was similar to the feeling I would get when I was a college and grad student after studying intensively

and taking long exams, except that it would happen at three P.M. without my having mentally exerted myself. In addition, reading, especially later in the day, became increasingly difficult, and I often had trouble remembering what I had read, sometimes even from one page to the next. In addition, I began to feel sometimes 'fuzzy' when I was in meetings, having little to add to discussions, particularly meetings held at the end of the day. I also noticed that I would often fall silent in group conversations, especially when they involved more complicated/controversial subjects, which had not been typical for me. I often felt I didn't have anything to add (the ideas just weren't there) or that my comment might not be on point because I hadn't completely followed the argument. Oftentimes when I did speak up, in a meeting or in conversation, I would formulate my comment in my head (which felt like work) and repeat it over and over until I spoke, just to make sure I said it right or that I didn't forget what I was going to say. This was not how I used to function."

3. *Decreasing interest in reading, an inability to follow or engage in complex conversations, and an inability to follow movies with complicated plots.* Conversations "became tiresome for me," Eleanor said. "I didn't know why. I had trouble following some that were not in my field and just wanted to close my eyes."

4. *Decreasing ability to recall what she read or heard.* "It felt exhausting to have to try to remember things, whether it was what to get at the supermarket or what kind of sushi my kids wanted to order," she said. The year before she began the ReCODE protocol, Eleanor told me, material she needed to read for a course "seemed very dense and I had no recall. I also had difficulty remembering other things I had

read, like novels or magazines. Reading (which I used to crave!) was no longer a pleasure."

5. *Decreasing vocabulary.* Eleanor struggled to find the right word, and began using a simpler vocabulary. "I might say *aggressive*, but had stopped saying *pugnacious* or *truculent*. I would say someone was 'thinking about something over and over' instead of saying that he was *perseverating* on something. I would say someone was very *social*, but I wouldn't say she was *gregarious*. Along these lines, I would also do word searches when speaking, where I might pause looking for the right word. I'd usually come up with a 'decent' word, or find a roundabout way to say something. For example, I would say that someone 'went about something following step by step like they should' because I couldn't access the word *systematic* to say *systematic approach*. This was disconcerting to me, and would take real mental effort, but it was not so obvious to be noticed by others. After about five to six months on the protocol, when I was talking to people, I would notice I would naturally use words that I hadn't used in many years—like those above—and it would surprise me because I had even forgotten that they existed."

6. *Mixing up words.* "It was not unusual for me to mix up my kids' names from time to time. But what started to happen shortly before I made my appointment with the clinic was that I would use words that were completely wrong. For example, while I was taking my kids to school, I called out to the tollbooth operator—loudly and confidently—'Conference call!' instead of *car pool*, to get my car pool discount. On another occasion, I called for my dog in the yard, yelling 'Chili!' (what I was making for dinner) instead of Juno (her name)."

7. *Decreasing processing speed.* She both thought more slowly, feeling "fuzzy" during work meetings in particular, and typed more slowly, as if the signals from her brain to her fingers had to travel through molasses.

8. *Increasing anxiety about driving and finding her way.* The many things drivers need to see and process, from the position and motion of other vehicles to the meaning of traffic signals and the movement of pedestrians, caused Eleanor such extreme stress that she felt she could barely operate the car.

9. *Difficulty remembering her to-do list and appointments; often feeling "overwhelmed" by what needed to get done.* Eleanor had started missing appointments and "was becoming very anxious and stressed about not being able to keep track of everything going on in my life," she said. "I used Google calendar and had reminders everywhere, but was still forgetting things. When I was younger, I used to be so confident in my memory. I never missed appointments and memorized phone numbers the first time I dialed them."

10. *Sleep disruption.* "I would awaken easily, and when I did, I would have great difficulty falling back to sleep; sometimes it would take hours. I would also awaken many, many times per night."

11. *No longer getting a mental boost from caffeine.*

12. *Trouble speaking the foreign languages, including Chinese and Russian, that she had once been proficient in.*

It typically takes many years, even a decade or two, for symptoms like these to become severe enough to qualify for a diagnosis of Alzheimer's disease, as Eleanor's case showed.

Nine years after the onset of these symptoms, when she was

age 49, Eleanor tested positive for the inherited risk factor for Alzheimer's, the gene ApoE4. She underwent neuropsychological testing, which revealed abnormalities consistent with her symptoms. In other words, Eleanor had not simply been experiencing "senior moments." Her brain was beginning to fail her. Besides the discrete symptoms she described, what did Eleanor feel during this bleak period? Because she recovered her ability to think, remember, and function, Eleanor is in an unusual position. She is like an explorer who ventured into a terrifying land from which few others had gotten out alive . . . but managed to come back, able to tell the rest of us what it was like. Here is how Eleanor described it to me:

> I want to articulate what it felt like to be in the "fog" of early cognitive decline—something I feel I have a special perspective on because I climbed out of it. I came up with the analogy of the feeling you get when you are wearing headphones and trying to talk to someone next to you. It sounds muffled and you feel more distant from others. Similarly, before I reversed, it felt like I had a filmlike gauze over my brain that kept me from really connecting with others and from being able to easily engage in normal conversational back-and-forths. It was sometimes an enormous effort to formulate my response, such as in work meetings, and then to convey it (without forgetting what I had wanted to say). It was as if that "gauze" were a barrier I had to punch through to get the thought out. Conversation, especially about more sophisticated topics, had become far from the effortless activity it had been when I was younger.

Eleanor began the ReCODE protocol in early 2015, and within six months noticed clear improvements in her cognition. She underwent neuropsychological testing after nine months, which confirmed the improvement: her feeling that she was back to normal was no figment of her imagination or of wishful thinking. It was real, it was quantified, and it was objectively measured. One month before those tests, in October 2015, here is how Eleanor described her feeling of returning to normal:

> I feel like I have had an awakening. I noticed a few improvements in August, but by September it was clear to me that a "fog" had lifted and I could identify specific changes in my cognitive functioning. I feel like my life is back, and I am writing to thank you and to share with you what I have experienced and learned in the event that my doing so might also help you in your research.
>
> Seeing these changes in myself has given me insight into what happened to my dad as well as into what was happening to me. I had been attributing a lot of things to "fatigue" or "age" but now I see that that wasn't true.
>
> 1. *Facial blindness.* I am now significantly better at recognizing people and remembering that I had met them. I noticed this in September, when I attended Parents Day at my kids' school. Usually that day makes me very anxious because I don't remember whom I know, whom I've met, and am just not sure who people are without name tags. This year I recognized all sorts of people, remembered their names and their kids' names, and knew little things about them. Even more, I had the confidence to say their names because I KNEW I knew them!
> 2. *"4:00 Fatigue."* That has gone away!! I see now that my father experienced this exact change in his late forties. He cut his days shorter at the hospital where he worked,

and zoned out with TV after three P.M. every day at home. We thought he was just exhausted from work. Now I know it was early dementia. You can't see this when you are in it.

3 and 4. *Reading comprehension and recollection.* Improved! Now when I read something or someone tells me something, I remember a lot of it—a big change for me. Now I can remain engaged and even follow conversations that are not in my field.

5 and 6. *Vocabulary and word search.* I find I am now using more words to describe things. I hadn't realized that my vocabulary had become limited and my speech less sophisticated, but it had. I see this now that I am starting to use "big" words again. I still search for words, but much less often, and now I actually find them!

7. *Clarity and thinking speed.* I am significantly sharper when helping my kids with essays and homework. I wrote one piece recently . . . something I haven't done in years . . . with speed and focus, similar to when I was younger. My typing speed is back, too.

8. *Driving.* The anxiety I had about driving is starting to let up.

9. *Appointments and to-do lists.* I recall appointments better now and the stress from the constant fear of missing things is abating. It's not perfect, but definitely improved. It takes much less effort to remember something. I no longer ask my kids to leave written messages whenever they ask me to do something for them.

10. *Sleep.* I did notice an improvement with my sleep when I started taking melatonin and magnesium in the evenings, at the outset of the protocol. I found that my first sleep stretch felt deeper, and lasted for three to four

hours (longer than it had), and that on some nights my awakenings didn't last as long, or happen as often. I do not feel "tired all of the time" anymore, and when I've had decent sleep, I feel great!

11. *Caffeine.* When I drink coffee, I feel an alertness I had stopped feeling.

12. *Foreign languages.* Surprisingly, the Chinese and Russian that I had not used in years started to come streaming back, and at one point I started writing down each word that reappeared.

One of the things that most strikes me about all of this is that I couldn't have told anyone that all these things were problems last year. I couldn't put it all together. I was functioning on the outside. I just thought things were sometimes "fuzzy," but couldn't identify specific problems. The changes come on slowly so that you don't really notice, and the mental fatigue is *so* powerful, it makes you think you are just exhausted or burned out. Now that I am improving, I can see the deficits for what they were. I feel like it is an "awakening" and just hope it lasts. I don't know how to thank you enough. Your protocol has truly changed my life.

No one would deliberately put herself in the condition Eleanor endured, yet we do it every single day just by eating the standard American diet and living the standard American life. The next chapter explains how.

CHAPTER 4

How to Give Yourself Alzheimer's: A Primer

Patient: Doctor, it hurts when I do <u>this</u>.
Doctor: Then don't do that.

WHY WOULD YOU want to give yourself Alzheimer's disease?! In truth, of course, you probably wouldn't, but looking at the multitude of factors that can contribute to the development and progression of Alzheimer's disease helps you to understand how to prevent the process in the first place, or reverse it once symptoms appear. It also gives you a checklist to see just how many of these factors you already have in your life.

Okay, how shall we start? Well, if you're like me, you often work late and find yourself craving a late-night snack, preferably something sugary, making your insulin level skyrocket right before bed, keeping it high while you're sleeping. Maybe you get to bed well after midnight and sleep poorly because of sleep apnea (often the result of weight gain). Nonetheless, you rise bright and early, getting just a few hours of sleep. Your feet have barely hit the bedroom floor when you start feeling stress as you contemplate the day ahead. You grab a typical Western breakfast—a sweet roll or doughnut, a large glass of orange juice, a big slug of low-fat milk in your coffee—and thereby get a hefty dose of inflammation-triggering dairy, take another step toward insulin resistance with the sugar, and poke holes in your gastrointestinal lining with the gluten. You pop your proton pump inhibitor to prevent gastric reflux, even though by reducing stomach acid you'll impair your ability to absorb key nutrients such as zinc and magnesium and vitamin B_{12}; then you'll take your statin, a great way to lower your cholesterol below 150 and thereby increase your risk for brain atrophy. Oh, and we'll do all this less than twelve hours after our late-night snack, which means the body never gets to induce autophagy and remove the accumulating amyloid and various damaged protein debris.

Rushing out the door keeps our stress level high, producing the cortisol that damages our hippocampal neurons. Next we'll jump in the car, making sure not to get any exercise before work and minimizing sun exposure, an excellent way to keep vitamin D levels suboptimal. Since we're stressed out and irritable from lack of sleep, we'll keep our interpersonal interactions high-pressured and unpleasant, avoiding positive social interaction and killing joy. When our blood sugar crashes around midmorning, we'll hit the office kitchen, where a thoughtful colleague has left a box of chocolate-chip muffins for everyone to partake of. Then lunch?! There's no time for anything but a sandwich from the cafeteria or deli—white bread, spongy saline-injected turkey with hormones and full of antibiotics and stress factors—yum! Alternatively, how about some mercury-laden tuna?! The salad doesn't look that good, anyway. Wash it down with a diet cola, to damage our microbiome. Now let's go for the brownie, so we can get our trans fats and minimize our healthful omega-3 fats.

At this point, we've done a yeoman's job of setting our physiological course for Alzheimer's disease. But if we want to get there even faster, we top it off with a cigarette, decreasing the delivery of oxygen to our tissues—that would include brain tissue—and sending hundreds of toxic chemicals into our bloodstream. No need to brush our teeth or floss—who cares that poor oral hygiene promotes systemic inflammation and destroys the barriers that otherwise keep bacteria such as *P. gingivalis* out of the brain?

Our postprandial torpor sends us to the vending machine and—hey, we worked so hard today, we deserve a treat!—to that luscious Frappuccino we've been keeping in the fridge. Sugar-and-fat runs have been our only "exercise" today (and every day), but who has time to get up and move around frequently? Finally it's time to hit the motorway, heading home while screaming at the idiot riding his brakes in front of us, thus keeping our blood pressure up and making our blood-brain barrier as porous as the colander we plan to use for tonight's gluten-filled pasta dinner. On second thought, let's get something from the takeaway. Start with large fries, a perfect source of Alzheimer's-inducing advanced glycation end products, or AGE—trans fats, starchy insulin, oxidized reheated oils with little vitamin E, and neurotoxic acrylamide. You can almost picture each fry with tiny little boxing gloves, snarling, "Let me at that hippocampus!" Add the burger— slathered in high-fructose corn syrupy ketchup, on a bun so packed with gluten it's the perfect way to punch holes in your intestinal lining and your blood-brain barrier.

Home again! Ignore that mouldy smell. Collapse in front of your favourite screen for some Netflix bingeing or other favourite fare, as long as it doesn't offer mental or physical stimulation. (Leave the Wii tennis and football to the kids.) Then we can top off the perfect Alzheimer's-inducing day with a relaxing margarita or three to accompany that amaretto cheesecake, then dutifully pretend to get caught up on work before drifting off to sleep with the lights on and the electronics still blaring. Rinse and repeat.

As you have no doubt surmised, the Alzheimer's-inducing lifestyle is horrifyingly similar to the lives so many of us lead. Don't panic, however: just as it takes many years for mild cognitive problems like Eleanor's to spiral into full-blown Alzheimer's, so it takes many years for the metabolic and other brain assaults that come from a typical Western diet and lifestyle to wreak their havoc.

That's the good news.

The bad news is that the more you see yourself in the lifestyle I described, the more certain you can be that it is already impairing your mental sharpness and that you already have one or more of the three neurothreats (inflammation, shortage of brain-supporting molecules, or exposure to toxic substances) that the brain responds to with what we now know as Alzheimer's, including by producing the sticky amyloid plaques that destroy brain synapses.

That is why ReCODE targets this treacherous triad. If you can eliminate these threats by changing the way you live, then the brain will not be pushed to produce the amyloid that we associate with Alzheimer's disease. Think of it as barring terrorists from getting on the plane: if airport security manages that, then passengers never have to fight the terrorists in the aisle of the 747. You want to keep neuroterrorists far, far away from your brain.

There is a tremendous amount you can do to achieve this on your own. For some parts of the protocol, such as identifying which of the triad of neuroterrorists your brain is (unbeknownst to you) already trying to fend off, it helps to work with a doctor and, in many cases, a health coach so you can arrange to get lab tests, optimize your programme, and track your response.

As noted above, cognitive decline is largely a matter of three fundamental threats to our brain: inflammation; a shortage of brain-boosting nutrients, hormones, and other cognition-supporting molecules; and toxic exposure. What we call Alzheimer's disease is a protective response to these three brain threats. Two of the threats, inflammation and a shortage of cognition-supporting molecules, are intimately linked to metabolism. Metabolism in turn is a function of our diet, our level of activity, our genes, and our exposure to and handling of stress. Since diet, activity, and stress also affect cardiovascular health and other aspects of our well-being, brain health is closely related to general health. No wonder so many of the conditions that increase our risk for Alzheimer's disease—from prediabetes and obesity to vitamin D deficiency and a sedentary lifestyle—are the result of what and how much we eat and exercise.

The good news is that although there are dozens and dozens of factors that can cause inflammation, a shortage of brain-supporting molecules, and susceptibility to toxic compounds, and thereby contribute to cognitive decline, they are all identifiable and all addressable—the sooner, the better. Here are the basics for addressing each neurothreat:

1. *Prevent and reduce inflammation.*

Inflammation is your body's response to attack, whether by infectious agents such as *Borrelia* (Lyme disease) or noninfectious stresses such as sugar-damaged proteins or trans fats.

We are constantly exposed to potential invaders, from viruses and bacteria to fungi and parasites. When we fight these pathogens, one of the ways we do so is by activating the immune system.

When the immune system floods the zone, so to speak, with white blood cells that engulf and devour pathogens, that's part of the inflammatory process. But while we need to mount an inflammatory response to fight acute threats (that redness around a cut is inflammation, and your white blood cells are fending off possible infection), if the threat is chronic and the inflammatory response is continuously activated, it's a problem.

Part of the way the body responds to invading pathogens is by producing amyloid, the very substance that forms the brain plaques that characterize Alzheimer's disease.[1,2] Furthermore, when you look inside the brain of someone who died with Alzheimer's disease, you find pathogens: bacteria from the mouth, moulds from the nose, viruses such as *Herpes* from the lips, *Borrelia* (the Lyme disease organism) from a tick bite. More and more scientific evidence is pointing to the conclusion that after a brain is invaded by pathogens, it produces amyloid, a potent pathogen fighter but one that eventually goes overboard, killing the very synapses and brain cells the amyloid was called up to protect.

Therefore, to prevent and reverse cognitive decline, you must address potential infections, optimize your immune system's ability to destroy pathogens, and reduce the chronic inflammation that results from fighting these organisms for years.

Inflammation can also arise without infection. It is triggered when we eat trans fats, for example, the artificial fats that were once ubiquitous in baked goods and fast foods (but are now being phased out), or sugar. The body also mounts an inflammatory response when damage to the intestines, often from consuming gluten or dairy or grains, causes "leaky gut." (See the box opposite for a list of foods with high gluten contents—all of which are to be avoided as much as possible.) In this condition, the gastrointestinal tract develops microscopic holes, allowing fragments of food or bacteria into our bloodstream. That too triggers

Foods containing gluten

(from the website of Dr. David Perlmutter,
http://www.drperlmutter.com/eat/foods-that-contain-gluten/)

- Wheat
- Wheat germ
- Rye
- Barley
- Bulgur

- Couscous
- Graham flour (whole meal flour)
- Kamut matzo
- Semolina
- Spelt

The following foods often contain gluten

- Malt/malt flavouring
- Soups
- Commercial stocks and stock cubes
- Charcuterie (ham, salami, etc.)
- French fries (often dusted with flour before freezing)
- Processed cheese (e.g., Dairylea)
- Mayonnaise
- Ketchup
- Malt vinegar
- Soy sauce and teriyaki sauces
- Salad dressings
- Imitation crab meat, bacon, etc.
- Egg substitute
- Tabbouleh
- Sausage
- Non-dairy creamer
- Fried vegetables/tempura
- Gravy
- Marinades
- Tinned baked beans
- Cereals
- Commercially prepared chocolate milk
- Breaded foods
- Fruit fillings and puddings

- Hot dogs
- Ice cream
- Root beer
- Energy bars
- Trail mix
- Syrups
- Seitan (wheat gluten)
- Wheatgrass
- Instant hot drinks
- Flavoured coffees and teas
- Blue cheeses
- Vodka
- Wine coolers
- Meatballs, meat loaf
- Communion wafers
- Veggie burgers
- Roasted nuts
- Beer
- Oats (unless certified gluten-free)
- Oat bran (unless certified gluten-free)

inflammation: the immune system recognizes these fragments of food, thinks they're foreign invaders, and attacks.

Chronic inflammation can arise when we are continuously exposed to dangerous microbes (such as when mouth bacteria keep leaking into the bloodstream, typically from damaged gums) or when we regularly ingest inflammation-triggering foods such as sugar. That's why ReCODE aims to roll back chronic inflammation by eliminating both ongoing infections and inflammation-inducing foods.

When the inflammation is caused by sugar toxicity, it is typically accompanied by insulin resistance, something that most

Britons, as well as over a billion people around the world, suffer from. We humans evolved to handle only small amounts of sugars (about 15 grams per day, less than half the amount in a 330ml soft drink). Sugar is like fire, a source of energy but very dangerous. If you have a fireplace in your home, the amount of wood and the size of fire needed to heat it depends on the size of the house: less wood/smaller fire if your house is small, more wood/bigger fire if your house is large. Now imagine that you shrink your house by 90 per cent, which is essentially what happens when we move less, as is true of sedentary-living Britons: we need less energy. That makes your fireplace effectively ten times as large. If you kept pouring on the wood and stoking the fire, your house would quickly become unbearably hot, the fire might escape from the fireplace, and you would do everything possible to keep your house from burning down. This is the stress most of us are now experiencing. Our bodies recognize sugar as poisonous, and therefore rapidly activate multiple mechanisms to reduce its concentration in our blood and tissues. For one thing, we store the extra energy as fat, which produces brain-damaging factors called adipokines.

But that still leaves our bloodstream awash in sugar—specifically, glucose. The glucose molecules attach to many proteins, inhibiting their functioning just as egregiously as if an octopus attached itself to a pole vaulter. Our cells respond to the flood of glucose by increasing the production of insulin, which reduces the glucose by, among other strategies, pushing it into cells. But your body, faced with chronically high insulin levels, simply turns down the response, and you become resistant to the effects of insulin.

And insulin is intimately related to Alzheimer's disease, by several mechanisms. For example, after insulin molecules do their job and lower the glucose, the body must degrade the insulin in order to prevent dropping the blood glucose too low. It does this via an enzyme called insulin-degrading enzyme (IDE). Guess what else IDE degrades? Amyloid, the protein fragment in the sticky, synapse-destroying plaques in Alzheimer's disease. But the enzyme can't do both at once. If IDE is breaking down insulin, it can't break down amyloid, any more than a firefighter can battle a blaze at the north end of town if he/she is raining water down on a conflagration at the south end. By diverting IDE from destroying amyloid, chronically high levels of insulin increase the risk for Alzheimer's disease.

Therefore, a critical part of ReCODE is reducing insulin resistance, restoring insulin sensitivity, and reducing glucose levels, thereby restoring optimal metabolism.

2. *Optimize hormones, trophic factors, and nutrients.*

When we eliminate inflammation by reducing chronic infections and insulin resistance, we remove threats that allow amyloid to accumulate. That thwarts brain damage. It's also crucial to give the brain a boost. The more you can strengthen your synapses, the harder it will be for any amyloid plaques that develop to destroy them.

That became crystal clear from a study presented at the annual meeting of the Society for Neuroscience in late 2016. Scientists analyzed the brains of people who died in their nineties and who had retained excellent memory until then. Some of the brains were riddled with amyloid plaques. Somehow, apparently, the brains of these nonagenarians were immune to the synapse- and memory-destroying effect of amyloid. How can that be? Follow-up studies continue, but there are two leading hypotheses. One is that if people are well educated and intellectually engaged throughout life, they may have enough redundant synapses to withstand the loss of some to amyloid plaques. Alternatively, it may be that some biochemical mechanism either fights amyloid, perhaps detoxifying it so it no longer destroys synapses, or strengthens synapses enough to withstand the amyloid assault.

I am all in favour of doing everything you can to increase your cognitive reserve. But I am also in favour of harnessing those bio-chemical mechanisms to make synapses as resistant as possible to the ravages of amyloid. To function at its best, your brain needs neuron- and synapse-supporting factors, including certain hor-mones, trophic factors, and nutrients. ReCODE offers ways to boost them. Among the synapse-strengthening compounds are brain-derived neurotrophic factor (BDNF), which can be increased through exercise; hormones such as oestradiol and testosterone, which can be optimized through prescriptions or via dietary supple-ments; and nutrients such as vitamin D and folate. Interestingly, when the brain runs low on synapse- and neuron-boosting com-pounds such as BDNF, it responds by producing—you guessed it—amyloid. You can begin to see the list of contributors to amy-loid production and cognitive decline—in other words, to Alzhei-mer's disease—growing, from the many processes inducing inflammation to insulin resistance to hormonal loss to reduced vitamin D to reduced BDNF (and related neurotrophic factors) to loss of other critical supporting nutrients and factors. We need to measure and address them all if we are to maximize our chances of reversing cognitive decline.

3. *Eliminate toxins.*

If a snake bites you and injects you with venom, you want an antivenin that will bind to the venom and inactivate it. Amyloid, it turns out, plays that role when the brain is infiltrated by toxic metals such as copper and mercury, or by biotoxins such as the mycotoxins produced by moulds. By binding up these toxins, amyloid keeps them from damaging neurons. Again, since it is crucial to prevent the formation of amyloid plaques, ReCODE offers an effective way to reduce toxic induction of amyloid, starting with the identification of the toxic exposure, removal of the source, and then detoxification that includes, among other things, detoxifying foods such as cruciferous vegetables, pure-water hydration, sauna-based removal of a specific class of toxins, and increasing critical molecules such as glutathione. That way, the brain has no reason to churn out amyloid.

AFTER DOING ALL you can to eliminate the three neurothreats of inflammation, shortage of synaptic support, and toxic exposure, it is crucial to restore lost synapses and protect new and remaining ones. Again, research from multiple groups has identified compounds that enhance synapse formation, as I explain in detail later.

You may have noticed that the programme I've just summarized is completely different from a prescription for a drug. Complex chronic illnesses such as Alzheimer's disease have many contributors, which is why their optimal treatment involves addressing all of the contributors—a personalized programme, not simply a pill. ReCODE is not only more comprehensive than taking a pill. It is also more effective. It is not a silver bullet targeted to a single abnormality; it is *silver buckshot* targeted to the multiple contributors to cognitive decline.

PART TWO

Deconstructing Alzheimer's

CHAPTER 5

Wit's End: From Bedside to Bench and Back

It is a riddle wrapped in a mystery inside an enigma;
but perhaps there is a key.
—SIR WINSTON CHURCHILL,
SPEAKING ABOUT RUSSIA IN 1939

To ME, THERE is nothing more fascinating than the workings of the human brain, and our journey from watching brain cells that had been growing in a lab dish disintegrate to the absolute joy of watching desperate and hopeless people flourish once again, returning to work and to their families' open arms, is a Sherlock Holmesian odyssey, ongoing and endlessly revealing. However, not everyone finds the death of a microscopic cell compelling, so while reading this chapter you might find your eyelids becoming heavy—descriptions of scientific research can be soporific, to be sure. My wife, an excellent family GP but not particularly interested in basic research, occasionally has difficulty falling asleep, and sometimes when she does I start telling her what I consider to be the most exciting current scientific research results. Within a minute, she is usually fast asleep, and I am left talking to myself. . . .

In this chapter I describe the scientific basis of Alzheimer's disease—the model that my colleagues and I have developed over three decades of research into the basic mechanisms of neurodegeneration and the biological rationale for ReCODE. Bits and pieces of these discoveries are contained in our more than 200 scientific papers. Like my wife, you may wish to skip this chapter and the next and go straight to the clinical assessment and treatment (chapters 7 to 11). But who knows, if you stay for the science, you just might find it interesting. . . .

Near the end of my freshman year at the California Institute of Technology, I ran across an enthralling book called *The Machinery of the Brain*, by physicist and engineer Dean Wooldridge.* Just a few months earlier, I had been surfing in Hawaii with my friends from the Greenback Surf Club. But now I had left the aquamarine roar of surf spots Kewalo Basin and shark-favourite Incinerators for the scientific epicentre, Caltech, where some of the most brilliant minds on Earth plumb the mysteries of black holes and dark matter, of molecular genetics and split-brain psychophysiology, in the process winning thirty-five Nobel prizes and, of course, serving as the setting of the television hit *The Big Bang Theory*. Wooldridge and Caltech opened my eyes—to insects with hardwired behaviour but no ability to reason, to the physiology of electroshock therapy, to the strange phenomenon of two sides of the brain thinking independently, like two beings in a single head! It was fascinating, and I got hooked on the brain—for life.

---

* Wooldridge is best known as the W in the pioneering aerospace and electronics firm TRW.

In the 1970s biologist Seymour Benzer, one of my favourite professors, had used *Drosophila*—the tiny fruit flies that swarm overripe bananas in our kitchens—to identify the actual genes that underlie behaviour. It was amazing! He was actually able to pinpoint a *Drosophila* gene required for learning and memory (the first such one discovered). Mutant flies lacking this gene were christened *dunce*, just one example of molecular biologists' habit of conferring memorable names to the genes and mutants they discover. Benzer discovered another gene that made fruit flies sleep all day and stay up all night, one that made males great at mating (called *savoir-faire*), one that left them with no idea how to court the ladies, another that produced gay fruit flies, and one that made the brain degenerate just like the brains of patients with Alzheimer's disease. Since Benzer was able to identify the single gene involved in each case, he could also identify the protein that each gene makes* and, through years of intense work, trace what each protein did, and where, in the flies' brains. That enabled him to work out the molecular mechanisms underlying learning and memory, diurnal rhythms (daily rhythms, timed by your internal clock), sexual behaviour, and many other functions of the fly brain.

At the time—this was the early 1970s—I was working in a chemistry lab, learning about triplet molecular states, quantum mechanics, and energy transfer. Although these topics may seem abstruse, they led to the following question: could we understand the most fundamental nature of brain diseases such as Alzheimer's disease, Parkinson's disease, and Lou Gehrig's disease, just as Benzer had revealed the genetic basis of behaviour with his dissection of *Drosophila* brain function, so that we might apply these

---

* Genes are made of four chemicals designated A, T, C, and G, which in various combinations code for the building blocks of proteins. Thus by discovering the genes and their spellings, Benzer was able to work out the protein that each gene made.

fundamental principles of chemistry to fashion the first effective treatments?

I realized something then: I needed to move from the research lab to medical school in order to learn about human brain diseases. I needed a deep understanding of what these neurodegenerative diseases—from Alzheimer's to Parkinson's to Lou Gehrig's and many more—do to their sufferers, what neuropathological changes occur in their brains, what the courses of the diseases look like, in order to gain insight into the fundamental mechanisms that drive these fearsome illnesses. If I were to have any hope of contributing to the discovery of effective treatments, I would need to learn more about these diseases.

It was the era of Dr. Marcus Welby, and medical schools were focusing on primary care. The country had fallen in love with the idea of the family practitioner, so people who wanted to use their medical degree to pursue biomedical research as well as treat patients were considered second-class applicants. One of the interviewers, a faculty member from an otherwise progressive university, told me I would be throwing my life away if I became a doctor instead of a scientist. When I argued that combining a knowledge of basic science with a sensitivity to patient needs could be an advantage for a doctor, he threw up his hands and said, "Okay, I just thought that maybe you wanted to make a difference in the world." As a naive 21-year-old, I was a bit shaken to hear that becoming a doctor would not allow me to "make a difference." Ironically, nine years later, after finishing medical school at Duke and doing a residency in internal medicine at Duke and a residency in neurology at the University of California, San Francisco, I received the book-ended criticism of being a "clinician wanting to do basic research."

One of the reasons I had chosen to do my neurology residency at UCSF in the first place was a young professor there named

Stanley Prusiner. Stan was studying a group of rare diseases called transmissible spongiform encephalopathies,* which, as the name implies, can be transferred from one brain to another, and which include diseases like mad cow disease. Stan went on to win the 1997 Nobel Prize in Physiology or Medicine for his discovery of prions, a term he coined to describe the agents—smaller than viruses and consisting only of protein without any genetic material—that cause these diseases.

After finishing a postdoctoral fellowship in neurodegenerative diseases in the Prusiner Laboratory, I established my own laboratory in 1989 at UCLA. I wanted to address two related questions that had motivated me from the outset. First, why do brain cells degenerate in diseases such as Alzheimer's? Second, is the underlying neurodegeneration mediated by developmentally related physiological signalling, or is it mediated by purely pathological nonphysiological processes? In other words, is Alzheimer's simply an accident, like dropping acid on your hand or being hit by a cosmic ray? Or is Alzheimer's disease something much more interesting, much more fundamental, something that reflects a change in the state of brain function? As the great physicist Richard Feynman said, "Nature uses only the longest threads to weave her patterns, so each small piece of her fabric reveals the organization of the entire tapestry." This is great news for physicists studying quarks. But would the threads of Alzheimer's disease reveal fundamental truths about the brain? And would they reveal a path to reverse the degenerative process?

The reason it is so critical to distinguish between these two possibilities—whether the neurodegenerative process is accidental

---

* The name reflects the fact that they are transmissible from one brain to another and make the brain so riddled with holes it looks like a sponge.

or programmed (meaning the result of normal brain physiology that has somehow been triggered in excess)—is that the treatments in each case would be entirely different. If neurodegeneration is akin to spilling acid in the brain, you would need to neutralize the acid, then think about using stem cells to repopulate the brain areas where the original neurons had been lost. If instead neurodegeneration is akin to activating an intrinsic brain programme—one that's also used for normal, healthy processes—then you would want to take a very different approach: you would want to understand this intrinsic programme in great detail in order to see where it has gone off the rails, reverse it, and return the brain to its healthy state.

Cell Suicide Is Painless, It Brings on Many Changes

When I set up my lab in 1989, there was no straightforward way to distinguish between these two possibilities for the simple reason that there was no simple model of neurodegenerative disease in a petri dish. That is, unlike taking cancer cells out of a patient in order to grow them in a lab dish and study their behaviour and vulnerabilities, you can't cut into a brain of a living person and scoop out some neurons. Furthermore, there was no way to measure the effects of Alzheimer's in a dish at that time. Therefore, in order to see exactly what causes synapses and neurons to be destroyed in neurodegenerative diseases such as Alzheimer's, we needed a way to grow neurons in a lab dish to re-enact the steps they go through that lead to the devastation of Alzheimer's. Such a neuronal cell culture would have to be genetically manipulable, meaning we could alter the genes in the neurons and see how that changed their behaviour and the course of the disease in a dish. And this in vitro model* would have to mimic the disease quite faithfully. Obviously neurons in vitro can't suffer or get lost in their own home or stare blankly at someone they've known for decades. But in theory they could go through the same degeneration as neurons in the brain of someone descending into Alzheimer's— much as oncology researchers have been able to grow malignant cells in vitro to track their progression and, crucially, their response to potential cancer drugs. We simply did not have such an in vitro model of neurodegeneration. In fact, there was widespread scepticism among neurologists in the early 1990s that such a model would be relevant. According to the conventional wisdom, any process that occurred in a few hours or days in a petri dish was unlikely to have any relationship to the processes that occurred over years in patients with neurodegenerative diseases. Fortunately, conventional wisdom turned out to be wrong, and what we discovered from the simple model we developed was what ultimately allowed us to develop the first effective protocol to reverse cognitive decline.

In 1994, my laboratory colleagues and I began growing rodent and human brain cells in petri dishes. (The human cells came from neuroblastomas or gliomas; such cancer cells grow and proliferate essentially forever, and thus are immensely useful sources of cell lines used in research. More recently, these have largely been replaced by stem cells, but stem cells were not available in 1994.) Using a process called transfection, we inserted genes linked to Alzheimer's and other neurodegenerative diseases into the cells and then observed them. Initially the cells looked unfazed, basically no different from cells that had not been transfected with disease-causing genes. But, surprisingly,

---

* *In vitro* means "in glass," and refers to where cells are growing or an experiment is taking place—in a lab dish or test tube. Its opposite is *in vivo*, meaning in a living organism such as a lab rat.

they would commit suicide at the drop of a hat! That is, when we disrupted the control cells by taking away some nutrients or adding any slightly toxic compound to the petri dish, they basically fought it off and hung in there. But when we made life difficult for cells containing genes for one or another neuro-degenerative disease, they all died, seemingly without putting up even the pretense of a fight! It was like an entire battalion surrendering after the enemy had fired off only a few rounds. Surprisingly, this was true across the board—whether the gene we slipped in was associated with Lou Gehrig's disease or Huntington's or Alzheimer's.

When we looked closely, however, we saw that the cells with Alzheimer's and other disease genes hadn't died the old-fashioned way. No. They had activated what's known as a suicide programme—a series of biochemical steps that kill the cell from within. It was cell biology's own Jonestown. To belabour the analogy, our battalion hadn't just surrendered after coming under attack; they had turned their weapons on themselves. The first time it happened, I was shocked and excited. We were seeing, for the very first time, the effects of a neurodegenerative disease not in a human brain over years, but in tiny cells in a dish—in a few days. This opened up all sorts of possibilities for asking what types of therapeutics might prevent or reverse the process.

Cellular suicide is a normal process when it occurs at the right place and time. For example, in the time it takes to count to two, a million of your white blood cells have committed suicide! And they have been replaced by a million new white blood cells. Such programmed cell death is critical for many of our bodily functions, and we would not be alive without it. Without cell suicide, we would have webbed fingers (since we would not lose the tissue between them), a brain that grows right out of the skull, and rampant cancers (because cells that become malignant would survive rather than commit suicide, as many actually do), along with many other problems. So cell suicide is crucial for life.

On the other hand, too much cell suicide, at the wrong place or the wrong time, causes birth defects and organ damage—and as this 1994 experiment showed, neurodegenerative diseases like Alzheimer's. The discovery that genes associated with Alzheimer's cause brain cells to become suicidal gave us just what we were looking for: a simple model to study Alzheimer's disease in a dish. Now we could ask what fundamental mechanisms drive the process and test potential treatments. Of course, anything we found would still need to be confirmed first in lab animals carrying human Alzheimer's genes (these are called transgenic mouse models of Alzheimer's disease) and, ultimately, in patients. But whereas discovering a single piece of the Alzheimer's puzzle in such lab animals takes about six months, in our cell culture we could make such discoveries in just a few days. This time frame gave us a wonderful opportunity to narrow down the myriad different possible mechanisms involved in Alzheimer's disease quickly, as well as to screen thousands of chemical compounds and identify those that block those disease-causing mechanisms.

Our First Eureka Moment

You have a remarkably powerful computer inside your skull. It contains an estimated 100 billion neurons, each with an average of almost 10,000 connections, for nearly one quadrillion—that's 1,000,000,000,000,000—total connections, or synapses, in your wonderful brain. Every feeling, every thought, every memory, every decision, every perfectly executed arabesque, every creation, every scam ever perpetrated, every tender act, every act of terrorism, every sin, and every act of human kindness—all originated in these connections, which is how brain cells communicate with one another. Every thought ever thought by a human being—Pontius Pilate's decision to send Jesus to Calvary, Julius Caesar's realization that even Brutus had turned against him, the choice you made at Starbucks yesterday and in the voting booth last election day—is the result of signals travelling down one neuron, crossing the synapse to the next neuron in a particular circuit, travelling down this neuron, on and on until you speak or move or otherwise give real-world expression to the activity inside your brain.

Each neuron in your brain needs a way to take in information from outside itself, in the space it occupies in the brain. To do that, neurons sport what are called receptors. These are protein molecules, made deep within the cell and then exported to its surface like a security camera being shipped from the factory to the home where it's to be installed. Receptors sense what is going on in the soup outside each cell (as well as inside), which is a caldron of molecular information. There are receptors that detect thyroid hormone and others for vitamin D, still others for oestradiol, for nerve growth factor, or for dopamine, the neurotransmitter associated with expecting rewards. Receptors sense molecules outside (or inside, depending on which receptor) the cell, grab hold of them the way the loading dock of a bakery pulls in delivery trucks packed with flour and sugar, and instruct the cell to respond accordingly, initiating a series of biochemical reactions inside the cell.* Each receptor does this billions of times each day; if they didn't, we would be lifeless blobs. So when we came upon a receptor in the basal forebrain, a brain area most affected in Alzheimer's disease, and had no idea what it was doing there, our curiosity was piqued.

---

* The process of responding to information outside a cell by initiating biochemical reactions inside a cell is called signal transduction.

We had hypothesized that it might be involved somehow in cell degeneration. We based this idea on its sequence of amino acids (amino acids are the chemical building blocks of proteins, kind of like the individual pearls on a necklace), but that notion was paradoxical because what little was known about its function was that it bound to (tightly interacted with) ligands called neurotrophins, which support brain cell *health* rather than death. A brilliant young UCLA undergraduate named Shahrooz Rabizadeh was working in my laboratory, and he placed the DNA for this gene—called p75NTR, the common neurotrophin receptor—into the neural cells, causing the receptor to be produced by the cells, and then added the neurotrophin ligand and quantified the resultant neural cell death. In December of 1992, he brought the data into my office and told me that the experiment had failed—the ligand-receptor combination had actually seemed to reduce the overall amount of cell death, not increase it.

Now, often the most interesting and revealing experiments—the moments when an invisible chemical or an inconsequential cell can move the Earth—are not the ones that succeed as expected, nor are they the ones that fail outright: they are the ones that yield results that are just the opposite of what you expected. In the Hegelian dialectic of thesis → antithesis → synthesis, such an unexpected and opposing result provides the very antithesis that is needed for the synthesis of new knowledge. And so it was for Shahrooz's results. When the neurotrophin ligand bound to its receptor, it did not activate the receptor to induce cell death, so our hypothesis was incorrect. But in a surprising twist, the receptor itself, *without* the ligand—the very state in which receptors are supposed to be idle—induced the cells to commit suicide! The cells that were supposed to be just fine—cells with an "inactive" receptor without the ligand—were committing suicide left and right. And even prior to the cell death, the synaptic connections would be lost.

But wait! The *ligand* that bound to p75NTR would *completely inactivate* the suicide mechanism—in essence, the ligand would talk the cell down off the ledge. Thus we had found a completely new type of receptor, one that was active in inducing cell death when receptors are supposed to be inactive—when awaiting ligand binding—and then flipped, preventing cell death when the ligand bound. This is something like finding a new type of lock that, as soon as the key (the ligand) is removed, burns down the house. What this meant was that once a cell produces this receptor, the cell becomes dependent on—literally addicted to—the ligand: the key must stay in the lock, or else. The consequences of producing this kind of receptor were, to the neuron, literally life and death. Once a neuron produces this receptor, it becomes dependent on the neurotrophin for its very survival: the neurotrophin key must stay in the receptor or the neuron dies. Therefore,

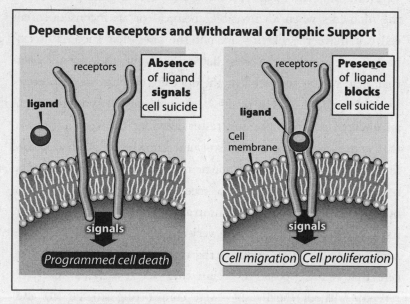

Figure 1. Dependence receptors induce cell death when they are not bound by their partner ligands, but this is turned off when the ligand binds the dependence receptor.

we dubbed these receptors dependence receptors, and published the result in the leading journal, *Science*.[1]

It was holiday season, and I spent hour after hour driving around in a daze thinking about these new receptors, foreign to everything I had been taught about receptor activation. I realized that the behavioural profile of such receptors suggested that they might be involved in the development of the embryo, in the development and spread of cancers, and in neurodegenerative diseases. That is exactly what turned out to be the case, and this gave us a new insight into Alzheimer's disease. Was it possible that the brain cells lost in Alzheimer's disease were triggered to die by dependence receptors that had lost their ligands?

The strength of any new theory lies in the accuracy of its predictions, its beauty in its simplicity, and its importance in the depth and breadth of its application. For the dependence receptor theory, it accurately predicts the molecular alterations in spreading cancer cells, offers a new method to treat the most serious complication of cancer—i.e., that it spreads throughout the body—and as you will see, offers us the first hint at how to treat Alzheimer's disease effectively. Its simplicity allows us to interpret a complicated set of observations in development, tumour invasion, metastasis, aging, and neurodegeneration, and thus its applicability is remarkably broad and far-reaching.

Twenty-one of these dependence receptors have now been identified, seven international meetings have been held, over a hundred papers have been published, and it has turned out that they control dependence on all sorts of different molecules, from trophic factors to hormones to anchoring molecules that hold cells in place. They do much more than control the spread of cancer. They control parts of the development of the embryo, the matching of inputs to targets in the nervous system, and the shrinkage of cells that occurs without the proper support. But we wanted to know if these receptors had anything to do with

Alzheimer's disease itself. If so, how do all of the pieces—from all of the more than 50,000 papers published on Alzheimer's disease—fit together?*

I could not help thinking back to something I had read as a first-year student in college. In 1928 Paul Dirac, who would win the 1933 Nobel Prize in Physics, wondered whether there might be something akin to an electron "hole"—that is to say, something that might be the opposite of the electron. His predicted particle—the antielectron, or positron—was discovered just a few years later, in 1932, proving the existence of antimatter. The dependence receptors we discovered on neurons sent their neurons "die!" messages whenever they were bereft of the neurotrophin molecules. The neurotrophins were therefore life-giving/death-preventing molecules. I wondered whether there might be a sort of anti-trophin. Theoretically, this would be a molecule that blocks neurotrophins from binding to the dependence receptor, perhaps because the anti-trophin itself has taken up residence in the receptor. (Back to our bakery analogy, the flour and sugar delivery truck can't get to the loading dock if the coal truck for the bakery's ovens is parked there.) If an anti-trophin were keeping neurotrophins out, the receptors would send the "die!" signal to the neuron just as if the neurotrophin were nowhere in the vicinity. To our surprise, we discovered that this is exactly what happens in Alzheimer's disease.

What Alzheimer's Disease Actually *Is*

As Dr. Aloysius Alzheimer himself observed, the brain of a patient with the disease that now bears his name displays plaques and tangles. The plaques, which resemble the spiky burrs of a

---

* Dependence receptors also turn out to play a role in tumour metastasis, in which cells break off from the primary tumour and spread to distant sites in the body.

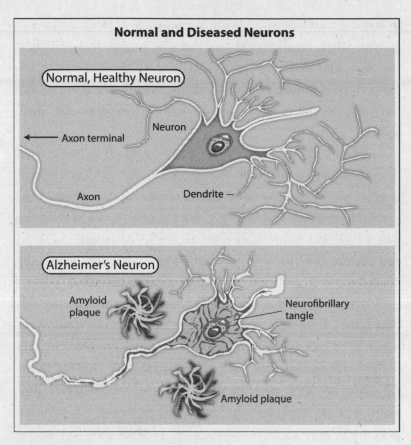

Figure 2. The brains of patients with Alzheimer's disease contain amyloid plaques and neurofibrillary tangles.

sweet gum tree, are, as I explained in chapter 1, made up largely of the peptide amyloid-beta (Aβ). The normal function of amyloid-beta continues to baffle neurologists, but somehow amyloid-beta is toxic to neurons, especially in the form of small gangs of amyloid-beta called oligomers. It turned out that amyloid-beta fulfils exactly the criteria you would want of an anti-trophin: it binds to multiple receptors on neurons, blocking the trophic signalling required to keep the dependence receptors from telling neurons to die.

Sometimes such trophic blocking is healthy. As I said above, in some circumstances cells are supposed to commit suicide—as when they are damaged or otherwise unable to fulfil their function, and therefore need to get out of the way and make room for replacements. But too much trophic blocking allows too many dependence receptors to send their neurons the "die!" signal.

A picture of what Alzheimer's disease actually *is* had started to take shape. A molecule, amyloid-beta, that acts as an anti-trophin accumulates at high concentrations in the brain, triggering dependence receptors to reduce connections (the synapses that are critical for memory and are lost in Alzheimer's disease) and ultimately kill the neurons. But what causes this oversupply of amyloid-beta?

To understand that, we needed to look at where amyloid-beta comes from—that is, the molecule it's made from. That molecule is called, rationally enough, amyloid precursor protein (APP). APP itself turned out to be a dependence receptor, as we discovered in 2000, and like the dependence receptors described above, it sticks out of neurons,* especially near synapses. APP is a good-sized receptor: it consists of 695 of those beadlike amino acids. (Amyloid-beta itself is only a small piece of APP, consisting of 40 or 42 amino acids). Exactly how APP functions as a dependence receptor offers further insight into the underlying cause of Alzheimer's disease.

After APP is produced by the neurons, it is cut by molecular scissors called proteases. The scissors cut at either three spots along APP's 695 amino acids, or at one distinct site. The different cut sites produce different fragments, of course, just as cutting the pasta coming out of your pasta machine *here* and *here* produces different kinds and lengths of pasta than if you cut it *there* and *there*.

---

* And, to a lesser extent, other cells.

In the case of APP, cutting it at three particular sites* produces four peptides: sAPPβ (pronounced soluble APP beta), Jcasp, C31, and amyloid-beta. All four of these peptides play roles in the processes that underlie Alzheimer's disease: loss of the brain's synapses, a sort of shrivelling up of the part of the neuron that

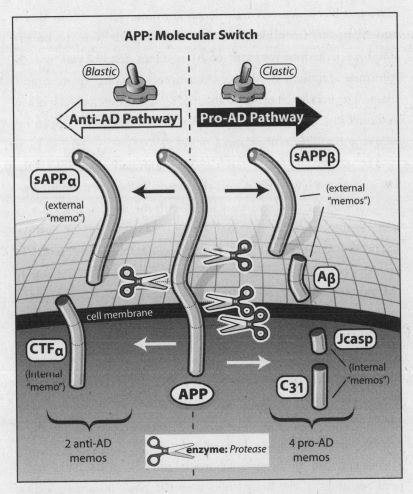

Figure 3. APP can be cut at one site, which produces two anti-Alzheimer's fragments, or at three different sites, which produces four pro-Alzheimer's fragments.

---

* They're called the β-site, the γ-site (gamma site), and the caspase site.

extends out to connect to other neurons, and the activation of neurons' suicide programme. On the other hand, APP can instead be cut at a single site. If this happens, the result is just two peptides: sAPPα and αCTF. This pair has effects completely opposite to those of the quartet above. They maintain synaptic connections, nourish the growth of neurons' reach-out-and-touch-someone fingers, and block neurons' suicide programme. They are, in short, anti-Alzheimer's peptides. I bet you have figured out the punch line here: to reduce your risk of Alzheimer's disease, you have to minimize production of the Alzheimer's-causing quartet and maximize production of the Alzheimer's-preventing duo. Obviously you can't just *will* this to happen. But you can make it happen by adopting the ReCODE protocol.

Let me repeat, for this is the very foundation of ReCODE. Depending on how APP is cut, the resulting fragments will support the cellular processes associated with memory formation and maintenance, such as the maintenance of synapses, or destroy them. As you might have guessed, *everyone with Alzheimer's disease* is on the wrong side of this crucial balance, with APP being cut in the way that produces the cognition-killing quartet. Just as important, everyone at risk for developing Alzheimer's disease is also on the wrong side. In their brains as well, APP is too often being cut so as to produce the devastating quartet rather than the cognition-supporting duo. It's just that in these brains the quartet has not been around long enough to wreak sufficient havoc to cause noticeable memory loss and cognitive decline. You can be sure, however, that—left unchecked—it will.

Being on the wrong side of a crucial physiological balance happens not only in the brain. It is also the basis of, among other diseases, osteoporosis, the loss of bone that is so devastating in the elderly (and especially common in women). In osteoporosis, there is an imbalance between bone formation, carried out by cells called osteoblasts, and bone resorption, due to cells called

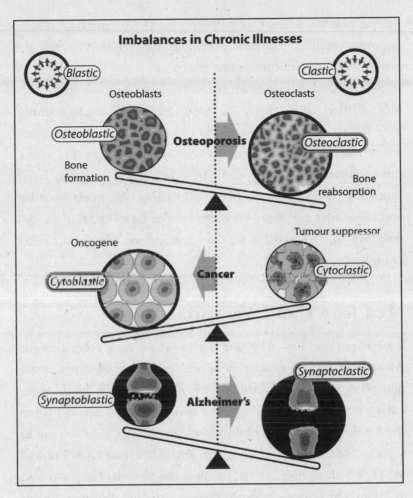

Figure 4. Imbalances in blastic (production) vs. clastic (resorption) signalling underlie chronic illnesses such as osteoporosis, cancer, and Alzheimer's disease.

osteoclasts. This is something like having two sets of home improvement contractors working for you, one that does demolition and the other that does construction. You can imagine what would happen if the first crew always showed up for work and did a thorough job with the sledgehammer, but the second contractor had to keep circling the block looking for a parking space. You would end up with less and less house. That's what happens in osteoporosis:

the osteoblastic activity is outpaced by the osteoclastic (bone-resorbing) activity. You lose bone, placing you at high risk for osteoporosis and life-threatening fractures.

We discovered that much the same thing happens in Alzheimer's disease. But instead of bone destruction overwhelming bone formation, synapse destruction (due to the destructive quartet) overwhelms synapse maintenance and formation (the job of the cognition-supporting duo). In other words, synaptoclastic signalling outpaces synaptoblastic signalling. We knew what we needed to find out next: what determines how much of the destructive quartet relative to, the constructive duo a particular brain has?

Mad Cows and Vampires

It turns out that how APP gets cut—at three sites, producing the Alzheimer's-causing quartet, or at one site, producing the neuron-nourishing duo—is determined by what molecule binds to it, among other things. If APP grabs a molecule called netrin-1 (from the Sanskrit word *netr*, meaning "one who guides"), APP is cut at a single site, thus producing the anti-Alzheimer's sAPPα and αCTF, which, as noted above, promote the growth of axons as well as all-around synaptic and neuronal health, and also prevent cell suicide.[2]

If, instead, APP grabs hold of amyloid-beta, APP is cut at the three sites, thus producing the Alzheimer's-causing quartet of molecules. That quartet includes, as you recall, amyloid-beta. Yes, when the amyloid-beta that comes from the cleavage of APP binds to APP, it pushes APP to make more amyloid-beta!

You may wonder where amyloid-beta came from in the first place. It sounds like a chicken-and-the-egg question: you need amyloid-beta to cause APP to be cut in a way that produces amyloid-beta. But remember that APP is a dependence receptor,

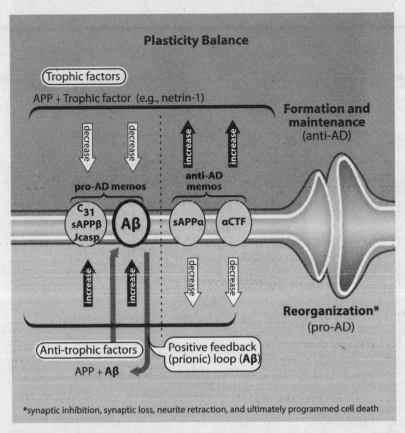

Figure 5. APP (amyloid precursor protein) can promote neurite growth and synaptic maintenance, thus supporting the formation and maintenance of memories; or the retraction of those projections, and thus the loss of memories. When netrin-1 binds APP, outgrowth occurs; when the Aβ peptide binds APP, retraction occurs.

so simply removing the trophic support, such as netrin-1, starts the ball rolling, causing APP to produce amyloid-beta.

The finding that amyloid-beta causes APP to make more amyloid-beta means that amyloid-beta is prionic. Just like the prions in mad cow disease, amyloid-beta can beget more of itself without the need for genetic material (which is how cells manufacture all other proteins). Like a tiny vampire, amyloid-beta bites the APP receptor and creates another tiny vampire. Together,

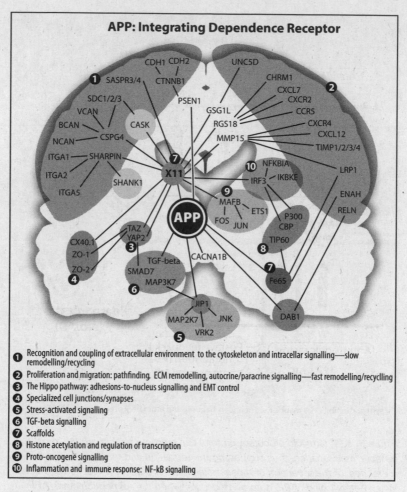

Figure 6. APP connectome. You can see that there are many different inputs involved in the balance that contributes to Alzheimer's disease.

APP and amyloid-beta create what's called a prionic loop, going around and around in a vicious circle, producing ever more synapse- and neuron-destroying amyloid-beta. This is why Re-CODE is designed to shift the APP balance back, reducing the cleavage that produces the amyloid-beta (the synaptoclastic cleavage) and increasing the cleavage that produces the two synaptoblastic peptides, sAPPα and αCTF.

Let me summarize quickly. Neurons sport receptors called APP. When APP grabs hold of a molecule called netrin-1, floating by in the intercellular environment, it sends a signal into the neuron that keeps the neuron healthy and functional. When APP fails to grab netrin-1 and lacks other trophic support, it defaults to a very different signal, telling the neuron to commit suicide. Grabbing hold of floating molecules has a second effect, however, this one on the APP itself: when the APP receptor grabs an amyloid-beta molecule, it unleashes a cascade of biochemical reactions that cause the APP to be cut in a way that produces more amyloid-beta. Amyloid-beta molecules begin to outnumber netrin-1 molecules. The APP receptor therefore is less and less likely to grab netrin-1 molecules and more likely to keep grabbing amyloid-beta. APP stops sending "stay alive and healthy!" signals into its neuron, ultimately causing the neuron and the synapses it has formed to die programmatically.

Any effective treatment for Alzheimer's should therefore include a method to shift the APP processing toward the synaptoblastic signals and away from the synaptoclastic signals.

In our next series of experiments, we searched for all the factors that might do this, not just netrin-1 and amyloid-beta. For it turns out that APP responds to—that is, it is affected directly or indirectly by—dozens of molecules. Crucially, all of them have been linked to Alzheimer's disease: oestrogen and testosterone, thyroid hormone and insulin, the inflammatory molecule NF-κB and the "longevity molecule" sirtuin SirT1 (famous for being activated by the resveratrol molecule contained in red wine), vitamin D . . . these and many others affect the APP receptor and whether it will be cut into Alzheimer's-causing or Alzheimer's-preventing snippets. So do sleep and stress and many, many other parameters.

Although these factors may seem unrelated, the reason they all contribute to the risk of Alzheimer's disease is that they exert leverage at the crux of the Alzheimer's pathway. Like Archimedes if he was given a place to stand and a lever long enough, these molecules and other factors can move the Earth, aka the pivotal point where APP is nudged down a pathway that destroys synapses and kills neurons or down a pathway that sustains and nourishes them.

If this all sounds complicated, well, it is. But what else would you expect of processes in the most sophisticated, complex system in the known universe—the human brain? In fact, however, it's not too different from what goes on in that bakery I keep referring to.

The bakery carefully monitors its revenue—from sales of biscuits and other products, from interest on its bank deposits, from renting out its space for the occasional party. It makes sure it has enough revenue to pay labour, materials, utilities, rent, and other costs. Does it have enough revenue to run the oven seven days a week or six? To pay three assistants or two? Does it have enough savings to remodel the old oven, install a new counter, tear out the old dropped ceiling in favour of something classier? Should it retire the old baker, who lately has been confusing Celsius and Fahrenheit on the oven settings?

So too does your brain continually evaluate what comes in and what goes out, what structures it has the resources to run, which can be replaced, which can be retired. It has nearly one quadrillion energy-demanding synapses to power. When it is time to form a new memory or learn a new skill, it must remodel some of those synapses or create whole new ones. That demands energy, raw materials, and brain activity, among other inputs. Each input has its own dependence receptor, which acts like an accountant, specializing in a single input: the testosterone receptor keeps track of how often it has been activated, the vitamin D receptor how often it has been, and other specialized receptors how often they have been. Each specialized accountant reports its status to APP, the chief financial officer. Thus we discovered that APP is actually a master dependence receptor, responding not to a single input, but rather integrating the inputs of many. APP adds them up to determine whether the income is sufficient to sustain the brain's far-flung synapses. If so, and there is room for continued remodelling and even expansion, then chief financial officer APP sends out two memos: that synapse- and neuron-sustaining duo, our old friends sAPPα and αCTF—and the brain is all systems go for synaptic maintenance and growth. But if our chief financial officer APP learns from the dependence receptors that they are not getting sufficient input, it sends out a different set of memos: the destructive quartet of sAPPβ, amyloid-beta, Jcasp, and C31. These molecules begin a campaign of synaptic downsizing in one or more brain regions.

When we are young, these two processes—synapse building/maintenance and synapse dismantling—are in dynamic equilibrium. When we learn, synapses are formed and strengthened. When we can afford to forget (what was the model of the car you passed right before getting home last night?), the synapses that once—often, as in the car example, very briefly—embodied that memory are broken up for parts, to be recycled into synapses encoding more important memories. The synapse-forming and synapse-destroying activities are balanced; we retain needed information and jettison the rest.

As we age, however, the inputs needed for synaptic growth and maintenance—hormones, nutrients, and more—grow more scarce. The receptors that sense them inform APP of this. The quartet of memos goes out: the brain's gargantuan network of synapses can no longer be sustained. It is time for strategic, well-coordinated downsizing.

That may sound like a terrible development—who welcomes the loss of neurons and synapses?—but in fact this downsizing is not inherently pathological. As my colleague Dr. Alexei Kurakin and I have written, Alzheimer's "disease" is, in many cases, actually an intrinsic downsizing programme for your brain's extensive and truly remarkable synaptic network. It is, in short, good for the brain—if you have a very expansive definition of "good." For what the brain is doing when, beset by Alzheimer's, it is downsizing is simple: it is pulling back, preserving only the functions it needs to stay alive, and not expending energy or resources on the formation of memories it doesn't need. Given a choice between remembering how to speak (or breathe, or regulate your body temperature) and remembering what happened on the *Friends* rerun last night, your brain opts for the former. And by extension, our most cherished, often-repeated programmes—our working skills, our favourite hobby skills—are often spared at the expense of new memories.

> WHEN NALA WAS 55, SHE BEGAN TO HAVE DIFFICULTY AT work. She developed a progressive dementia. A PET scan showed that her brain was riddled with amyloid, and genetic testing that she carried one copy of ApoE4 (the copy of the chromosome she inherited from her other parent was ApoE3). Both the amyloid and her ApoE status supported a diagnosis of Alzheimer's disease. An MRI showed that several brain regions had shrunk, as happens in the disease. Her score on the Montreal Cognitive Assessment (MoCA) screening test was only 6 out of 30, and on some days it was 0. Nala was unable to remember, to dress, shower, brush her hair, go to the bathroom by herself, or do any other activities of daily living. Yet she retained her ability to play the piano exquisitely.

And that is the condition we call Alzheimer's disease. To anyone suffering from Alzheimer's, of course, it is small comfort to know that the brain made a deliberate "choice" to preserve life-sustaining functions at the expense of the abilities—remembering and thinking, understanding and imagining—that make us human. But that's what happens. If your APP chief financial officer receives information from the dependence receptors that there are not enough hormones and vitamins and nutrients and other synapse- and neuron-sustaining molecules to maintain existing synapses and form new ones (for new memories), then APP sends out its synaptic-downsizing memos. As in corporations that follow a "last in, first out" philosophy of layoffs, recent memories go first, older ones next, and the oldest ones last. Thus Alzheimer's patients often remember their childhood of eighty years ago better than the breakfast they had an hour ago. Synapses controlling vital functions such as breathing are typically spared. And then, at last and mercifully, comes death.

The realization that dozens of molecules affect APP, and therefore the chances that you'll develop Alzheimer's, did more than lay the groundwork for ReCODE. It also explained why single drugs—approved and experimental—have failed repeatedly to stop, let alone reverse, the cognitive decline of Alzheimer's. The reason is that drug companies have been like roofers called to a home that had been pummelled with baseball-sized hail. The storm left dozens of holes in the roof, which the home-owners would like fixed. Yet the roofers fixated on a single hole. They may have done a bang-up job of slathering that hole with roofing tar, keeping rain from pouring in. Unfortunately, they did nothing about the other thirty-five holes, and the home is filling up with so much rainwater the owners are looking up specs for an ark.

I give the example of thirty-six holes because research in my lab has identified thirty-six different contributors to whether APP goes down the Alzheimer's-causing or Alzheimer's-preventing pathway. These explain all of the risk of Alzheimer's, at least as far as it has been measured in studies of large populations. So while there may turn out to be a few more than thirty-six, as mentioned

A Roof with 36 Holes

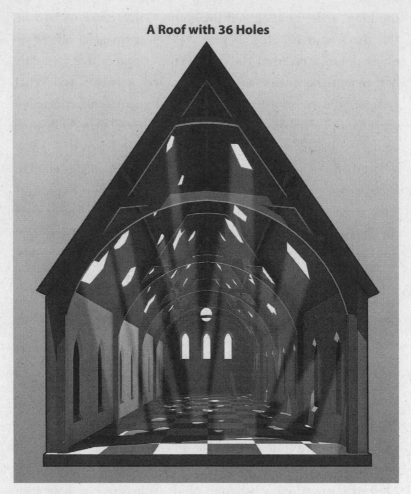

Figure 7. Thirty-six holes in the roof. There are at least thirty-six different mechanisms contributing to Alzheimer's disease pathophysiology, so fixing just one has little chance for success. The laboratory results reveal the size of each hole for each person.

above, it is likely that there are not too many more—certainly not hundreds.

Crucially, the prionic loop has a practical implication for how we understand and address these thirty-six factors. There is a threshold that needs to be reached in order to tip the balance toward APP's anti-Alzheimer's pathway. What this means is that you don't have to address all thirty-six holes. When you have patched enough of them, the rest aren't serious enough to let much water into your house. If we leave our roofing analogy to get back to Alzheimer's, the presence of a few of the factors nudging APP down the Alzheimer's-causing pathway isn't enough to exert that nudge in enough of your brain neurons enough of the time to cause Alzheimer's. Unfortunately, we don't yet have a simple way to measure how many of the thirty-six each person can safely live with, and each hole is a different size for each person, depending on his/her genetics and biochemistry, so it's best to address as many as you can until you see improvement. This is in fact what happens in the treatment of cardiovascular disease. When you address enough of the key pathophysiological parameters, like lowering your blood levels of triglycerides and reaching a healthy weight, you reverse cardiovascular disease, eliminating arterial plaque, as Dr. Dean Ornish has shown. Even if you do not patch all of the cardiovascular holes—maybe you still have an imperfect diet or some mild stress—you can often reduce arterial plaque as long as the other parts of the programme are followed optimally.

The discovery that at least thirty-six factors affect whether the brain goes down a synapse-destroying pathway that ends in Alzheimer's disease or a synapse-preserving pathway that reverses cognitive decline and maintains brain health has one obvious implication: no single drug is optimal to keep the brain on the healthy pathway, let alone steer it there after it has started down the Alzheimer's pathway. Why? Such a drug would have to do all of the following:

- Reduce APPβ-cleavage
- Reduce γ-cleavage
- Increase α-cleavage
- Reduce caspase-6 cleavage

- Reduce caspase-3 cleavage
- Prevent amyloid-beta oligomerization
- Increase neprilysin
- Increase IDE (insulin-degrading enzyme)
- Increase microglial clearance of Aβ
- Increase autophagy
- Increase BDNF (brain-derived neurotrophic factor)
- Increase NGF (nerve growth factor)
- Increase netrin-1
- Increase ADNP (activity-dependent neuroprotective protein)
- Increase VIP (vasoactive intestinal peptide)
- Reduce homocysteine
- Increase PP2A (protein phosphatase 2A) activity
- Reduce phospho-tau
- Increase phagocytosis index
- Increase insulin sensitivity
- Enhance leptin sensitivity
- Improve axoplasmic transport
- Enhance mitochondrial function and biogenesis
- Reduce oxidative damage and optimize ROS (reactive oxygen species) production
- Enhance cholinergic neurotransmission
- Increase synaptoblastic signalling
- Reduce synaptoclastic signalling
- Improve LTP (long-term potentiation)
- Optimize oestradiol
- Optimize progesterone
- Optimize E2:P (oestradiol to progesterone) ratio
- Optimize free T3
- Optimize free T4
- Optimize TSH (thyroid-stimulating hormone)
- Optimize pregnenolone
- Optimize testosterone

- Optimize cortisol
- Optimize DHEA (dehydroepiandrosterone)
- Optimize insulin secretion and signalling
- Activate PPAR-γ (peroxisome proliferator-activated receptor gamma)
- Reduce inflammation
- Increase resolvins
- Enhance detoxification
- Improve vascularization
- Increase cAMP (cyclic adenosine monophosphate)
- Increase glutathione
- Provide synaptic components
- Optimize all metals
- Increase GABA (gamma-aminobutyric acid)
- Increase vitamin D signalling
- Increase SirT1 (silent information regulator T1)
- Reduce NF-κB (nuclear factor kappa-light-chain-enhancer of activated B cells)
- Increase telomere length
- Reduce glial scarring
- Enhance stem-cell-mediated brain repair

And even this list may not be exhaustive. As you can see, this is a very tall order for a single drug. Combining medications (experimental or FDA approved) with a comprehensive programme actually makes sense from a mechanistic standpoint, and might allow some drug candidates to succeed in clinical trials when they otherwise would have failed. That is, a typical drug will address one or a few of the items on the list above. If dozens of other Alzheimer's-causing processes go unaddressed, of course monotherapy will fail. Our discoveries about the multiple factors affecting the plasticity balance demonstrated conclusively that that was not the way to go. On the other hand, combining a programme like ReCODE with a drug candidate may well allow the candidate to succeed in trials in which it might otherwise have failed.

Drug Addiction

Screw the FDA, I'm gonna be DOA.
—Matthew McConaughey in *Dallas Buyers Club*

By 2000, our research had begun to suggest that there is a critical balance in the making and storing of memories. We called this the plasticity balance because it appears to mediate critical processes involved in memory formation. One side of the balance supports memory formation and maintenance, whereas the other side supports forgetting through the reorganization of synapses.

Our research showed that everyone with Alzheimer's disease is on the wrong side of this plasticity balance: their brains are pulling back synapses faster than they are forming them, destroying synapses crucial to memory. Our research also showed that when we shifted this plasticity balance toward the "good" side, which we did genetically in a mouse with "Mouzheimer's" disease, the mouse's memory improved markedly, as shown by its ability to remember where submerged platforms inside a pool are located (and therefore where it needs to swim in order to get out of the water).[3]

We therefore searched for drug candidates that shift this balance toward the good side, the memory side. In 2010 we discovered one called tropisetron.[4] This drug is typically given to cancer patients so that chemotherapy does not make them nauseated, but it turns out that the way it works—basically, by blocking serotonin receptors in the brain, while simultaneously activating cholinergic receptors critical for memory, interacting with APP, and reducing inflammation—alleviated some of the memory loss in the mice. When we compared tropisetron to the commonly used Alzheimer's drugs in our Mouzheimer's mice, it proved to be superior,[5] leading us to begin the application process to perform a clinical trial—a human study—of tropisetron.

I was enthusiastic about tropisetron, but I realized that a major problem might complicate the trial. In the Mouzheimer's mouse, the Alzheimer's produced is simple. It is due to a mutation in APP, and so is unlike 99 per cent of human cases of Alzheimer's. The pathology, in particular amyloid plaques and loss of synapses, is there, but the root cause is very different. This limits the usefulness and even the relevance of the standard mouse model of Alzheimer's disease. That's because in people, unlike mice, there are many contributors to Alzheimer's disease—that is why I tell patients to imagine a roof with thirty-six holes, and understand that it may take patching many of them to bring about the optimal effect. Tropisetron blocks four[6] of the thirty-six contributors we knew about at the time. That's wonderful for a drug, but still far short of optimal; after all, the other thirty-two factors could still be contributing to Alzheimer's disease.

In 2011 we therefore proposed the first comprehensive trial for Alzheimer's disease. Instead of a single pill, we proposed that we combine tropisetron with the forerunner of ReCODE: a comprehensive programme of nutrition, exercise, synapse-supporting supplements, hormonal optimization, specific herbs, sleep optimization, and stress reduction, all aimed at shifting the brain's balance from synapse destruction to synapse preservation by removing the contributors (inflammation, shortage of trophic factors, toxic compounds) that trigger the brain's over-the-top (and ultimately, Alzheimer's-causing) defences.

Why did we not try to test a single drug? By this time, we had a good sense of how many "holes" would have to be patched—how many molecules the brain needed more of or less, how many brain processes needed to be revved up or quieted down—in order to treat Alzheimer's disease: at least thirty-six. However, just to be sure, our 2011 proposed trial included a group that was treated with tropisetron alone, so that we could compare this with the programme, as well as a combination of the two.

How do you go from watching cells die under a microscope to helping someone reverse his or her cognitive decline? How do you go from forgetful fruit flies or furry Mouzheimer's patients to humans who desperately want to stay with their loving families? Well, if you are developing a single drug, there is a well-worn path. First you conduct preclinical (animal) studies. Then if those show that the experimental drug might work, you ask the Food and Drug Administration in the US or the appropriate government regulatory body in the UK to give you approval for human clinical trials. You start with Phase 1, to test the drug's safety in a small number of volunteers (usually healthy people, but sometimes patients). If the drug seems safe, you move on to a Phase 2 clinical trial, which tests efficacy in a small number of patient volunteers. If it still seems safe and shows hints of working against the disease, you launch a Phase 3 clinical trial with, often, hundreds if not thousands of patients. If you're really lucky, the Food and Drug Administration (or regulatory body) approves the drug and it starts being sold. Developing a new drug takes years, if not decades, and costs an estimated $2.5 billion.

Unfortunately, what we were discovering about Alzheimer's disease made it impossible to even try to follow this playbook. By 2011 we had discovered that no fewer than thirty-six molecular mechanisms contribute to Alzheimer's.

We therefore decided to test the single drug, tropisetron, alone or in combination with the programme we came to call ReCODE. What I was most enthusiastic about was that the proposed trial would allow us to dissect how much of the effect was due to the drug, how much was due to the programme, and whether the two were synergistic, making the combination more effective than the sum of the effects of each alone. This was to be accomplished simply by including four arms (groups of patients) in the study: one with placebo, one with drug (tropisetron), one with the programme and placebo, and one with both the programme and tropisetron. We had proposed that the trial be performed in Australia, where tropisetron is available (it is also available in forty-eight other countries, but not the United States nor the UK where it was discontinued in 2008). We eagerly awaited approval from the institutional review boards (IRBs) that approve human trials.

What came back, unfortunately, was the beginning of a perfect storm of rejection.

The IRBs denied us permission to conduct the trial. In the opinion of the scientists and physicians who sat on the IRB, we didn't understand how to performme a clinical trial, since we were suggesting a programme rather than a single pill. Clinical trials, they insisted, are designed to test a single variable, usually a drug or procedure, but we were suggesting testing multiple components simultaneously. Our counterargument, of course, was that they didn't understand Alzheimer's, because it is not a single-cause disease but one with many potential contributors. It makes no more sense to try to treat Alzheimer's disease with a single agent than it does to treat a roof with thirty-six holes with a single patch of roofing compound. (Ironically, some of the doctors who sat on the IRBs expressed interest in using the protocol with their patients, despite their refusal to allow us to run the trial.)

When it rains, it pours, right? As soon as the IRBs turned us down, my colleagues and I received an angry note from a philanthropist who had supported our research, telling us that, if we had been his employees, he would have fired us for failing to convince the IRBs to allow our trial. But it did not end there: we had applied to a prominent Alzheimer's foundation for support for this first comprehensive trial for Alzheimer's disease. They turned us down, too, saying they did not "see the rationale for the inclusion of [our protocol, which] is of uncertain relationship to the study drug." Of all of the thousands of applications for funding to that foundation, here was their reviewer, faced with the one protocol that was actually going to work—the needle in the haystack—and he could not see it. He could not consider the possibility that the repeated failure of single drugs might be due to the need for complementation with a multicomponent programme that would address the *many* underlying contributors to Alzheimer's. (The foundation ended up giving the support we had requested to another group, for a trial of yet another monotherapy. You guessed it: the drug failed.)

During this struggle I could not help thinking about the birth of functional medicine, in which a doctor determines the root causes of illnesses and treats all contributing factors. Drs. Jeffrey Bland, David Jones, David Perlmutter, Mark Hyman—starting about two decades ago—began treating complex chronic problems like type 2 diabetes, lupus, and obesity with unprecedented success. Yet medical schools had virtually no interest in teaching about this approach. As the pioneers of functional medicine discovered, you know you are doing something that is paradigm changing when you are doing it right in front of everyone but no one can see it.

After this triple rejection—from the IRBs, the foundation, and the philanthropist—I was dejected. When your research takes you in a direction that goes against multibillion-dollar corporations, governmental juggernauts, indignant academic experts, solipsistic foundations, officious bureaucrats, overworked practitioners, and a global mind-set, I realized, the proverbial snowball in hell is laughing at your chances. But I kept in mind something the brilliant physicist Richard Feynman once said: "For a successful technology, reality must take precedence over public relations, for Nature cannot be fooled." It is the underlying mechanisms of a disease that dictate what treatment will ultimately prove to be efficacious—not the drug companies, not the government, not the reviewers, not the NIH, not the foundations, not the billionaires. Those are the groups that dictate which treatments will be *tested*, but not which will prove effective.

Shortly after these setbacks, I received a call, asking if I would speak with someone who was having problems. It was Patient Zero.

The standard avenues by which scientific discoveries become medical therapies had failed us—and had failed Alzheimer's patients. The clinical trial system is just not set up to test a comprehensive programme like ReCODE. But the bench research had pointed us in the right direction, showing us that a personalized, targeted, precision medicine approach to Alzheimer's disease makes far more sense than a one-size-fits-all, monotherapy approach. This allowed us to come up with the ReCODE programme and show that it works to reverse cognitive decline in Alzheimer's disease and the pre-Alzheimer's conditions MCI and SCI.

These clinical successes did something else. The usual progression in biomedical research is from the lab to the clinic, from scientific research to medical treatments. But sometimes what we learn in the clinic informs our scientific understanding of a disease. That has been the case with ReCODE and Alzheimer's disease. As more and more patients have tried and succeeded with the programme, their experience has taught us a great deal. Most important, it has taught us that although no single compound can raise brain levels of synapse-supporting trophic factors, reduce inflammation, increase insulin sensitivity, and patch the other thirty-plus holes in the roof that contribute to Alzheimer's, we can patch them all with the right combination. It requires determining which of the thirty-six contributors a patient had and then tailoring a treatment regimen—a regimen based in large part on diet, exercise, sleep, stress reduction, and other lifestyle factors.

CHAPTER 6

The God Gene and the Three Types of Alzheimer's Disease

Man still bears in his bodily frame the indelible stamp of his lowly origin.

—CHARLES DARWIN

OKAY, IT'S TIME to take a deep breath! After twenty-eight years of suicidal cells and brain-shrink genes and confused fruit flies and forgetful transgenic mice, we have, for the first time, a rational molecular picture of what Alzheimer's disease actually *is*. Let's put it to the test: a key trial of any scientific explanation is how well it accounts for all of the facts. For Alzheimer's, the 800-pound fact in the room is that ApoE4 causes a person's risk of developing the disease to soar. Since ApoE4 is the strongest known genetic risk factor for Alzheimer's disease, does our explanation have a place for it? It does.

As I explained in chapter 5, Alzheimer's disease occurs when dependence receptors that reach out for hormones, vitamin D, brain-derived neurotrophic factor, and many other neuron- and

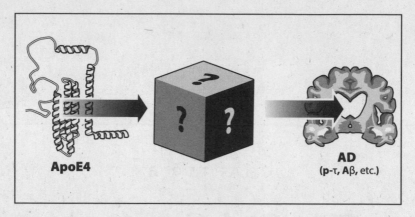

Figure 8. ApoE4 increases the risk for Alzheimer's disease—but how? What is in the black box between the ApoE4 allele and Alzheimer's disease?

synapse-supporting molecules come up empty (or emptier than is ideal), and then report that shortfall to APP. After taking in this news, APP reacts by sending out the four downsizing memos— the quartet of synapse- and neuron-destroying molecules. It turns out that ApoE4 increases how often APP sends out that downsizing quartet (rather than the two synapse- and neuron-supporting memos—that is to say, molecules).

How does ApoE4 promote the production of the devastating quartet and suppress the promotion of the healthy duo? Well before ApoE4 became implicated in Alzheimer's, researchers knew it carried particles of fat. Once ApoE4 became linked to Alzheimer's, the dogma became that ApoE4 reduces the clearance of the amyloid-beta peptides. Since amyloid-beta, as you recall, is part of the prion loop, the more it hangs around in the brain (that is, the less clearance), the more APP will churn out the devastating quartet (which includes amyloid-beta).

ApoE4 does indeed reduce the clearance of amyloid-beta peptides, but ApoE4 also does something even more fundamental, as we discovered. It also enters the nucleus and binds very efficiently to DNA, according to our studies led by Dr. Rammohan Rao, who is both an excellent researcher and an Ayurvedic doctor, geneticist

Dr. Veena Theendakara, and biophysicist Dr. Clare Peters-Libeu. This is something like discovering that your butcher—the guy who totes the fat—is also a senator involved in formulating the laws of the land. In fact, it has turned out that ApoE4 can bind to the upstream regions—called the promoters—of any of 1,700 different genes, thus reducing the production of the associated proteins. Since there are only about 20,000 genes in the human genome, and therefore in every cell, 1,700 is an impressive fraction of that total. No wonder ApoE4 is also involved in cardiovascular disease, inflammation, and more; through its effects on so many genes it can reprogramme cells!

That is only the start of ApoE4's talents. Among the others that are relevant to Alzheimer's:

- It shuts down the gene that makes SirT1, a molecule that has been linked to longevity and, as mentioned above, has an anti-Alzheimer's effect. (Resveratrol, a compound in red wine, *activates* the SirT1 protein.)
- It is associated with activation of NF-κB (nuclear factor kappa B), which promotes inflammation.

This is why ApoE4 is associated with a heightened inflammatory response: it quashes several different genes that limit inflammation, while turbo-charging the NF-κB that promotes it.

So let's sum up. This explanation of Alzheimer's disease tells us a lot:

1. Where Alzheimer's disease comes from and how it starts. It comes from a protective response to inflammatory insults (such as infections or trans fats), suboptimal nutrients, trophic factors, and/or hormone levels, or toxic compounds (including biotoxins, such as those from mould or bacteria) that cause the APP receptor—the long molecule that

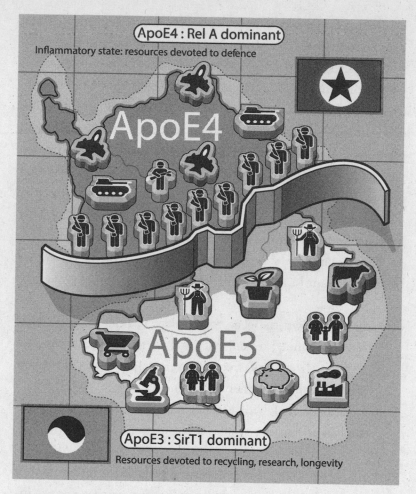

Figure 9. ApoE4 has a pro-inflammatory effect, activating the inflammatory factor NF-κB and thus committing cellular resources to protecting the cell from invaders. On the other hand, with ApoE3, the inflammatory response is less than with ApoE4, the system is SirT1 dominant rather than NF-κB dominant.

protrudes from neurons—to be cut into four fragments, including amyloid-beta, that downsize the neural network and eventually destroy synapses and neurons. When the APP molecule is cut into those four pieces, it is not cut into the two pieces that nourish and maintain synapses.

2. Its inner workings. Alzheimer's disease is a state of the brain in which there is an imbalance between the reorganization of synapses that have outlived their usefulness and which the brain can stand to lose—healthy destruction—and the maintenance or creation of existing and new synapses, respectively, which the brain needs to sustain old memories and form new ones (as well as perform other cognitive functions). That imbalance comes from too many of the synapse- and neuron-destroying quartet of molecules snipped from APP and too few of the synapse- and neuron-sustaining duo of molecules snipped from APP, as described above.

3. How to give yourself Alzheimer's. Live your life in a way that keeps your brain supplied with as many as possible of the thirty-six factors that influence whether APP gets cut into the destructive quartet or the beneficial duo.

4. How to prevent it. Live your life in a way that minimizes the number of the thirty-six inducing factors in your brain. This is described in detail in chapters 8 and 9.

5. Why more than 99 per cent of the pivotal trials of experimental Alzheimer's drugs have failed. They targeted only one of the thirty-six contributors to the disease.

6. How to stop the process leading to Alzheimer's if it has already begun. Evaluate your genetic and biochemical status to determine where you stand (as described in chapter 7), then address each identified contributor, as described in chapters 8 and 9.

7. How to reverse Alzheimer's if it has already taken hold. Evaluate your genetic and biochemical status to determine where you stand (as described in chapter 7), then address each identified contributor, as described in chapters 8 and 9.

This research has delivered one more big dividend. It has shown that Alzheimer's disease is not a single disease but is actually three distinguishable syndromes.

This new understanding of Alzheimer's—that it is the result of a programmed campaign of synaptic and neuronal downsizing, in response to too few molecules that cause the dependence receptor APP to be cut in a way that supports neuronal and synaptic health—offers us, for the first time, the ability to reverse the process. It tells us that simply reducing amyloid-beta, as drug companies have spent billions of dollars trying to do, is unlikely to help unless we also identify and remove the *inducers* of the amyloid production. Simply removing amyloid represents the equivalent of tearing up a single one of the four downsizing memos. Although that might delay the downsizing slightly, the other three memos have still gone out, and the brain is acting on them. More important, tearing up one memo does not address the root cause of the problem, just the response to it.

Now it's time to turn to the first step in the ReCODE protocol: determining which of the three types of Alzheimer's disease you have or are at risk for. This will allow you to fashion the optimal personalized programme to minimize your risk and, if you are already experiencing cognitive decline, get back to optimal function. The first step toward doing that is determining which of the three major subtypes of Alzheimer's or its precursors you're dealing with: hot, or inflammatory; cold, or atrophic; vile, or toxic.

TYPE 1 IS inflammatory (hot). It occurs more often in people who carry one or two ApoE4 alleles and therefore tends to run in families. And it shows how Alzheimer's disease is woven into our very existence as humans. Five to seven million years ago, our arboreal forebears, the common ancestor of chimps and our own lineage *Homo*, underwent a relatively small number of DNA changes, or mutations, that resulted in the lineage leading to modern humans. Surprisingly, these mutations included genes associated with inflammation—the very process linked to cardiovascular disease, arthritis, and many other ailments, not to mention aging itself. (Inflammation is the process that so many of us try to counteract with fish oil, baby aspirin, or anti-inflammatory diets.) Why would so many of the very genes that distinguish us from our primate cousins—that, in other words, make us distinctly human—turn out to promote inflammation? Good question.

Caleb "Tuck" Finch, a professor of the neurobiology of aging at the University of Southern California, thinks he may have an answer. Tuck noted that when our ancestors became bipedal, descending from the trees and walking the savannah, inflammation was actually an advantage. Inflammation, which as noted earlier is part of the reaction by the immune system to foreign invaders, allowed our ancestors to survive stepping on dung, puncturing their feet, eating raw meat filled with pathogens, and sustaining wounds during hunts as well as while fighting with each other. In all of these situations, mounting a robust inflammatory response protects against life-threatening infection.

As we age, however, inflammation promotes cardiovascular disease, arthritis, and other woes—including Alzheimer's disease. This trade-off is called antagonistic pleiotropy, in which a genetic alteration enhances fitness early in life at the expense of longevity. Arguably the most important of all of the inflammatory genes that were affected in our leap from chimpness to humanness is ApoE. From the dawn of humankind until relatively recently, ApoE came in only one "flavour," or allele, called epsilon 4, or ApoE4. For millions of years, therefore, we all carried two copies of ApoE4, one inherited from each parent—the very state that puts us at very high risk for Alzheimer's disease. Of course, since we do not have preserved brains from these protohumans, we have no way of knowing whether many of them actually developed Alzheimer's disease; however, it is unlikely, in part because few lived long enough and in part because their lifestyles actually covered many of the thirty-six holes—they led much less sedentary lives, ingested far fewer simple carbohydrates, had no processed foods, and had much less toxic exposure.

Then, just 220,000 years ago, a cosmic ray or chemical mutagen or simple random chance led to the appearance of ApoE3. If the mutation was in the genes of a lucky ovum or sperm, it was transmitted to offspring, and suddenly a whole different gene was swimming in the human gene pool. Another such mutation-causing event happened about 80,000 years ago, and for the first time someone—and eventually his or her progeny—was the happy bearer of yet another allele of the ApoE gene, called ApoE2.*

Today, most people carry two copies of ApoE3. This gives them a genetic risk of Alzheimer's of about 9 per cent. But 25 per cent of Americans, about 75 million, carry a single copy of ApoE4; they have a risk of Alzheimer's disease of about 30 per cent. And 7 million carry two copies of ApoE4, pushing their risk well above 50 per cent. That is, it is more likely than not that people who inherited an ApoE4 from both parents will develop Alzheimer's, and this is often, though not always, the inflammatory subtype.

This subtype typically begins with a loss of the ability to store new information, even as long-held memories and the ability to speak, calculate, spell, and write are retained. In people who carry two copies of ApoE4, symptoms often begin in the late forties or

---

* Scientists can date the appearance of mutations by counting how much they differ from what came before—in this case, ApoE3 and ApoE2 vs. ApoE4—and knowing, roughly, how many thousands of years it takes for that amount of change to occur.

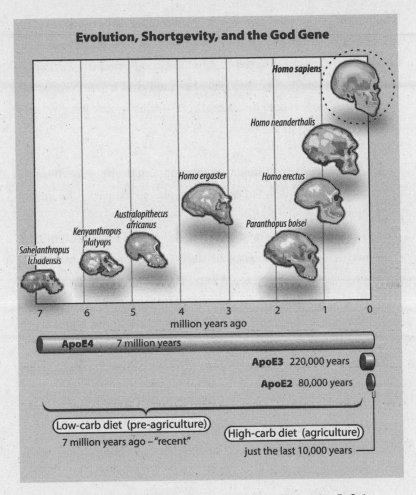

Figure 10. ApoE4 and human evolution. ApoE4 is our original ApoE. Only 220,000 years ago did ApoE3 appear, with ApoE2 emerging about 80,000 years ago.

fifties. For people who carry one copy of ApoE4, symptoms typically begin in the late fifties or sixties. For those with no copies of ApoE4, symptom onset is typically in the sixties to seventies. The hippocampus, which turns our experiences into long-term memory, loses volume, but most other brain regions don't, at least early in the process. The brain's temporal and parietal regions, which are responsible for many remarkable functions such as speech, calculation, recognition, and writing, use less glucose, an indication of reduced activity. Our detailed studies of patients with this form of Alzheimer's have revealed that it is accompanied by several telltale biochemical markers—which laboratory testing can assess:

1. An increase in C-reactive protein, made by your liver as part of an inflammatory response to threats like infections.

2. A decrease in the ratio of albumin (a key blood protein that acts as a rubbish collector, removing unwanted molecules such as amyloid and toxins and thus keeping the blood pristine) to globulin, a catchall name for some sixty blood proteins including antibodies. This ratio decreases when there is inflammation.

3. An increase in interleukin-6, which also rises with inflammation.

4. An increase in tumour necrosis factor, another protein whose levels rise in response to inflammation.

5. Accompanying metabolic and hormonal abnormalities such as insulin resistance.

Inflammatory Alzheimer's responds most quickly to the ReCODE protocol.

TYPE 2 IS atrophic (cold). This type also occurs more frequently in people who carry one or two copies of ApoE4, but typically initiates symptoms about a decade later than the inflammatory type. Like the inflammatory type, atrophic Alzheimer's also typically presents with the loss of ability to form new memories, even as the ability to speak, write, and calculate are retained.

There is no evidence of inflammation; inflammatory markers may actually be lower than normal. Instead, the overall support for brain synapses has dried up:

1. Levels of hormones including thyroid, adrenal, oestrogen, progesterone, testosterone, and pregnenolone are usually suboptimal.
2. Vitamin D is often reduced.
3. Insulin resistance may occur, or insulin levels may be too low.
4. Homocysteine may be high (although homocysteine may also be increased in type 1).

This type typically responds more slowly than the inflammatory type to treatment.

A 75-YEAR-OLD PSYCHIATRIST DEVELOPED SEVERE DIFFI-culty remembering new information, and this progressed over two years. She had no difficulty organizing, calculating, dressing, or speaking. She underwent a PET scan that showed typical findings for Alzheimer's disease. Her hippocampal volume was at only the 16th percentile, and her online cognitive assessment placed her at the 9th percentile for her age. She was ApoE4 negative (ApoE3/3). Her blood chemistries showed reductions in vitamin D, pregneno-lone, progesterone, oestradiol, free T3 (thyroid), and vitamin B_{12}, as well as increased homocysteine. A diagnosis of type 2 MCI (mild cognitive impairment, pre-Alzheimer's) was made.

She began on the ReCODE protocol, and over the ensuing twelve months, she noted marked improvement. Her cognitive assessment increased from the 9th percentile to the 97th percen-tile. Her significant other said that her memory went from "disas-trous" to "just plain lousy," and finally to "normal." Her follow-up labs showed improvements in vitamin D, pregnenolone, proges-terone, oestradiol, free T3, vitamin B_{12}, and homocysteine.

Alzheimer's types 1 and 2 sometime occur together. In this case, people have the inflammation characteristic of type 1 with the reduced support for brain synapses characteristic of type 2. One combination of types 1 and 2 is so common, it deserves its own type: type 1.5 is glycotoxic (sweet):

1. Glucose levels are chronically high, resulting in alteration to various proteins (called glycation) and in inflammation, as in type 1.
2. The high level of insulin secreted in response to the high glucose results in insulin resistance, so that insulin no longer works as well as a neurotrophic molecule, and this loss of trophic support is characteristic of type 2.
3. Types 1, 2, and their combination are all the result of the programme of downsizing that I described above, in which there is an imbalance between the production and destruction of synapses. In contrast, type 3 is very different, as described immediately below.

TYPE 3 IS toxic (vile). This subtype tends to occur in people who carry the common ApoE3 allele rather than ApoE4. Alzheimer's doesn't typically run in their families; if a relative did develop the disease, it usually occurred after age 80 or so. The toxic subtype strikes at a relatively young age, with symptoms typically beginning in the late forties to early sixties, often following great stress, and rather than beginning as memory loss, starts with cognitive difficulties involving numbers or speech or organizing. If types 1 and 2 represent strategic downsizing of an enterprise, with the brain destroying synapses faster than it creates them, then this third type is like tossing grenades into a building: everything is at risk. As a result, the patient loses not only recent memories but also old ones (and by *memory*, I mean not only episodic memory, the recollection of discrete facts and the events of your life, but also procedural memory, or how to do things both complex, like play bridge, and simple, like speak). People with this subtype of Alzheimer's often have difficulties with maths, struggling to calculate tips or figure out bills; with finding words; with spelling or reading. Psychiatric effects such as depression and attention deficits are also common.

MOLLY, A 52-YEAR-OLD WOMAN, PRESENTED WITH A TWO-year history of cognitive decline, which had started with difficulty with numbers: she found herself unable to figure a tip or pay bills, and then after several months she was forced to ask for help to write a grant proposal. Prior to the onset of her problems, she had had major life stresses with closing companies, family issues, job-related problems, and four episodes of anaesthesia, followed finally by entry into menopause. She declined rapidly and developed a simple, childlike affect. Despite this, she was able to learn and re-member the names of all twenty-eight children on the playground at her son's school. Family history was negative for dementia. Her MoCA (Montreal Cognitive Assessment) score was 19 out of 30, indicating significant impairment. Her MRI showed global cerebral volume loss, advanced for her age. There were several areas of FLAIR (fluid-attenuated inversion recovery) hyperintensity in the subcortical and periventricular white matter. In addition, there was atrophy of the cerebellum, a region of the brain typically spared in Alzheimer's disease. Despite this, her cerebrospinal fluid was diagnostic of Alzheimer's disease, since it showed an increased phospho-tau accompanied by a reduced Aβ42.

She was ApoE 3/3, hs-CRP was slightly high at 1.4, albumin: globulin ratio low at 1.57, hemoglobin A1c normal at 5.3 per cent, fasting insulin normal at 4.5, TSH slightly high at 2.14, free T3 normal at 4.2, free T4 normal at 1.0, progesterone low at < 0.21, oestradiol low at 3, 17-hydroxypregnenolone low at 14, morning cortisol 9, and vitamin D low at 22. Her serum copper was normal at 101, zinc very low at 56, and copper:zinc ratio high at 1.8:1. These results indicate that she had mild inflammation, along with likely adrenal fatigue, suboptimal thyroid function, and a low vitamin D. In addition, she had a markedly low zinc and high copper:zinc ratio.

These type 3 patients showed the poorest response to our original protocol of the three groups—and indeed, this was one of the important drivers for the development of the more sophisticated ReCODE protocol that we now use. Together with their very atypical presentation for Alzheimer's disease—virtually all had been assumed to have something other than Alzheimer's disease (e.g., frontotemporal dementia or vascular dementia) until the spinal fluid or PET scans forced a diagnosis of Alzheimer's disease upon the doctors—the question of what causes this unorthodox form of Alzheimer's disease became a crucial one, a mystery whose solution could impact millions of patients. What could be driving this disorderly form of Alzheimer's, this random, slovenly degeneration?

A fascinating clue appeared in the extensive blood tests, the very tests deemed unnecessary by health insurance groups and unimportant by most doctors. Many, although not all, of these patients with type 3 Alzheimer's disease had strikingly low zinc in their blood sera. In addition, many had triglyceride levels that were disproportionately low compared to their cholesterol levels. We discovered that this third type of Alzheimer's disease has its own characteristic biomarkers:

1. It affects many brain areas, not only or even predominantly the hippocampus, with MRIs showing that regions throughout the brain have atrophied (shrunk).

2. There is often neuroinflammation and vascular leak, as shown by a specific finding on MRI called FLAIR (fluid-attenuated inversion recovery), in which there are multiple abnormal small white spots on the MRI.

3. Often these patients have low zinc in the blood, high copper, and thus a high ratio of copper to zinc. That ratio should be about 1, with about 100mcg/dL each. But many patients

with this subtype 3 have serum zinc in the 50s, with copper as high as 170, and thus a ratio much higher than 1.

4. Patients with this subtype 3 are often diagnosed initially with something other than Alzheimer's disease, such as frontotemporal dementia or depression, or diagnosed as "atypical Alzheimer's," but the abnormal PET scans and spinal fluid (if a spinal tap is performed) show that they do indeed have a form of Alzheimer's.

5. Hormonal abnormalities, in which the system that responds to stress—the circuit consisting of the brain's hypothalamus, the pituitary gland at the base of the brain, and the adrenal glands atop the kidneys (together called the HPA axis)—is dysfunctional. This may show up in lab tests as low cortisol, high reverse T3 (a thyroid test), low free T3, low pregnenolone, low oestradiol, low testosterone, or other hormonal abnormalities.

6. High blood levels of toxic chemicals such as mercury or of mycotoxins, which are produced by moulds. Since mercury makes a beeline for tissues such as bone and brain, measuring its concentration in the blood isn't necessarily indicative of its presence. Therefore the assessment should use a chelating agent, which grabs on to mercury and pulls it out of the tissues. The level of mercury in the urine over the next six hours is often abnormally high, indicative of high mercury levels in the tissues.

Mainstream science holds that toxic chemicals are not a cause of Alzheimer's disease. The Alzheimer's Association says, for instance, that "according to the best available scientific evidence, there is no relationship between silver dental fillings and Alzheimer's." On the other hand, there are documented cases in which the removal of such amalgam fillings—which contain about 50 per cent mercury and 15 per cent tin in addition to the silver—has seemed to improve patients with Alzheimer's disease. To make matters more confusing, some epidemiological studies argue against a role for amalgam fillings as a risk factor for Alzheimer's, whereas others argue that exposure to mercury might indeed increase your risk of Alzheimer's disease.[1]

Is it possible that toxic compounds such as mercury play a role in at least some cases of "atypical" Alzheimer's disease, in which cognitive deficits like trouble speaking and calculating appear before memory loss? We've all heard of carcinogens, chemicals that can cause cancer, but are we also exposed to *dementogens*, which might cause cognitive decline? I began to call the spouses, significant others, and patients with this form of Alzheimer's. To my surprise, *all* had histories of toxic exposures. One had grown up in Toms River, New Jersey, where toxic chemicals secretly dumped by a local dye- and plastics factory reached families' water wells and were linked to a cluster of childhood cancers. Another had a sibling with childhood leukemia, which can be caused by exposure to toxic chemicals, and for years had worked for a chemical company where, he told me, he regularly inhaled strong chemical odours—and the compounds that caused them. Two other patients had lived in homes heavily contaminated with moulds. Another had worked with sewage, and several had had unusually extensive dental amalgam work.

Given what I had heard, I realized it might be important, in this group of patients, to perform sensitive tests for the detection of toxic chemicals, even though such tests are not typically done in the assessment of patients with suspected Alzheimer's disease.

KARL, 55, HAD HAD COGNITIVE COMPLAINTS FOR A YEAR, and they were getting worse. A numbers whiz his whole life, he now struggled to balance his cheque book. He had been a superb professional poker player, but now he couldn't remember the cards. He often used the wrong word, or a different word from that he wished to use, and found himself calling a person by the wrong name. He also had difficulty paying attention; watching a basketball game, he would forget which team had the ball. His thoughts sometimes raced, and he had bouts of mild depression. There was no family history of Alzheimer's disease.

A PET scan revealed a pattern typical of Alzheimer's disease, though mild at this stage. He was diagnosed with mild cognitive impairment, a precursor to Alzheimer's disease, and no further evaluation or treatment was suggested other than annual follow-up. He was later found to be ApoE4-negative (ApoE3/3).

When Karl contacted me, I suggested he undergo testing for heavy metals, including mercury, and for mycotoxins (toxins from moulds, such as aflatoxin, ochratoxin, gliotoxin, and trichothecenes). The lab found that Karl's mercury level was one of the highest they had recorded in years. Karl responded very well to treatment for his mercury toxicity. Not only did his overall cognition improve. So did his poker.

The three types of Alzheimer's disease correspond to the three processes that influence APP to send out the four downsizing memos: inflammation (type 1), loss of trophic support (type 2), and exposure to toxic compounds (type 3). This mirrors the three hats worn by the multi-talented molecule, amyloid-beta, which is derived from APP. It is part of the inflammatory response and can function as an antimicrobial agent (thus it is part of your body's ability to fight infections); it responds to inadequate levels of hormones, vitamins, nutrients, and other supportive (or trophic) factors by downsizing the more expendable synapses; it is part of the protective response to toxin exposure—for example, binding very tightly to metals such as mercury and copper.

These three different functions of amyloid-beta, and the different type of Alzheimer's disease associated with each, mean that removing amyloid-beta is likely to have very different effects on Alzheimer's disease, depending on the type a patient has. If amyloid-beta is removed from the brain of a patient with the

Table 1. Characteristics of type 3 Alzheimer's disease (from Bredesen, *Aging*, 2016, 3).

Characteristic	Comment
Symptoms begin before age 65.	Symptoms often begin in the fifties or late forties.
Usually ApoE4-negative.	Typically ApoE3/3.
No family history, or family history with symptoms beginning only at ages much older than the patient's.	The few with positive family histories are often those with ApoE4.
Symptoms often occur around the time of menopause or andropause.	Hormone status appears to be intimately related to type 3 Alzheimer's disease.
Depression precedes or accompanies the cognitive decline.	Depression is often associated with HPA axis (hypothalamic-pituitary-adrenal) hormonal dysfunction.
Headache is an early symptom, and sometimes the first.	Headache is a common feature in association with toxin exposure.
Memory consolidation is neither the initial nor the dominant symptom.	Typical symptoms include executive function deficits (planning, problem solving, organizing, focusing), inability to manipulate numbers/perform calculations, trouble speaking or loss of speech, problems with visual perception, or problems with learned programmes such as dressing.
Precipitation or exacerbation by great stress (e.g., loss of employment, divorce, family change) and sleep loss.	The degree of dysfunction is also markedly affected by stress and sleep loss.
Exposure to mycotoxins or metals (e.g., inorganic mercury via amalgams, or organic mercury via fish) or both.	Exposures can be evaluated by blood and urine tests.
Diagnosis of CIRS (chronic inflammatory response syndrome) with cognitive decline.	Cognitive decline is common with CIRS.
Imaging suggests brain changes not seen in most cases of Alzheimer's.	FDG-PET may show frontal as well as temporoparietal reductions in glucose utilization, even early in the course of the illness; MRI may show generalized shrinkage in the cerebral cortex and cerebellum, especially with mild FLAIR (fluid-attenuated inversion recovery) hyperintensity.

Characteristic	Comment
Low serum triglycerides or low ratio of triglycerides to total cholesterol.	Triglycerides are often in the 50s.
Low serum zinc (<75mcg/dL) or RBC zinc, or ratio of copper to zinc >1.3	Copper to zinc ratio should be 1.0, and values > 1.3 are associated with cognitive decline.
HPA axis dysfunction, with low pregnenolone, DHEA-S, and/or AM cortisol.	Hormonal abnormalities are common in this type of Alzheimer's disease.
High serum C4a, TGF-β1, or MMP9; or low serum MSH (melanocyte-stimulating hormone).	These tests indicate exposure to biotoxins such as mycotoxins.
HLA-DR/DQ associated with multiple biotoxin sensitivities or pathogen-specific sensitivity.	This genetic test indicates that you are particularly sensitive to biotoxins, and is positive in about 25 per cent of people.

inflammatory subtype, then if there are underlying microbes that are being fought by the inflammatory response, the removal of the amyloid could create further problems. If it is removed from the brain of someone with the atrophic subtype, there may theoretically be a delay in progression (a bit like firing the CFO and continuing to spend), but it may ultimately lead to a less orderly downsizing, thus losing critical cognitive abilities. These same concerns go for the patients with type 1.5, glycotoxic (sweet), since it is a combination of types 1 and 2. If amyloid is removed from the brain of a patient with the toxic subtype, this can be a significant problem if there is continued toxic exposure, since part of the protective response will have been lost.

The discovery of the three subtypes of Alzheimer's has crucial implications for practical therapeutics. To make a real difference to patients already in the grip of Alzheimer's or pre-Alzheimer's, and to keep at-risk people from developing it, we need to know which contributing factors to cognitive decline are present, and then address each one.

PART THREE

Evaluation and Personalized Therapeutics

CHAPTER 7

The "Cognoscopy"— Where Do You Stand?

Sometimes it takes a good fall to really know where you stand.
—HAYLEY WILLIAMS

W E ALL KNOW that when we turn 50, we should have a colonoscopy, an excellent way to catch premalignant lesions in the colon or rectum and thus prevent colorectal cancer. But what about your brain? The way for all of us over 45 years old to prevent cognitive decline is to have a "cognoscopy," evaluating all of the potential contributors and risk factors.

You can't fix a problem you're unaware of, so whether you are interested in preventing cognitive decline or reversing it, you first need to determine in detail where you stand in terms of your vulnerability to the three insults of inflammation, suboptimal hormones and other brain nutrients, and toxic compounds. Only then can you identify what needs to be addressed in order to improve cognitive function. The blood tests that will tell you this are increasingly available, although not all are available routinely on the NHS so you may have to seek out private practitioners and labs (more about this in Appendix A).

In people who have developed cognitive symptoms such as memory loss, ten to twenty-five laboratory values are often not optimal for brain function, while people who are at risk for cognitive impairment but not yet symptomatic typically have three to five suboptimal values.

Late in the progression of Alzheimer's, there is such a great loss of neurons and synapses that correcting the causes of those losses won't necessarily reverse cognitive decline. (We have seen some improvements recently in people with Montreal Cognitive Assessment [MoCA] scores as low as 1, which is very late in the course of Alzheimer's disease; these are the exceptions, however.) In such late cases, the cognitive horse has already fled the neurological barn. Thankfully, however, there is a relatively large window of opportunity not only to prevent but also to reverse Alzheimer's: during the asymptomatic phase, which may last a decade or so; during subjective cognitive impairment, which can also last a decade or so; during mild cognitive impairment, which may last several years; even during the mild to moderate phases of Alzheimer's. The earlier the causes of synapse loss and cognitive decline are identified and corrected, of course, the better your chance of avoiding full-blown Alzheimer's and even mild cognitive impairment, and more complete an improvement you can expect.

Before I go through each factor that we want to evaluate, let me contrast what I advise to how a patient with cognitive decline is usually evaluated. I'll quote the notes from a work-up by a well-known neurologist who specializes in Alzheimer's disease and practises at one of the US's most outstanding academic centres for Alzheimer's research and treatment: "MRI of the brain and blood for CBC (complete blood count), metabolic panel, thyroids, B_{12}. I asked the patient and his wife to keep an eye on his disabilities to manage money, medications, and transportation. I prescribed donepezil 5mg once per day."

This "gold standard" evaluation failed to include:

- *Genetics:* There was no information on the patient's ApoE status, or on dozens of other genes that raise the risk for Alzheimer's disease.
- *Inflammation:* This key player in Alzheimer's disease was not evaluated.
- *Infections:* Despite rapidly accumulating data implicating several different infections in Alzheimer's disease—such as *Herpes simplex*-1 virus, *Borrelia* (Lyme disease), *P. gingivalis* (an oral bacterium), various fungi, and others—no tests for any of these infections were performed.
- *Homocysteine:* This amino acid, which is causally associated with brain atrophy and Alzheimer's disease, was not measured.
- *Fasting insulin level:* This critical biomarker of the insulin resistance that occurs in Alzheimer's disease was not even mentioned.
- *Hormonal status:* Levels of hormones crucial for optimal brain function were not assessed; although thyroid function was checked, the key thyroid tests weren't done.
- *Toxic exposure:* Neither mercury nor mycotoxins were tested.
- *Immune system:* The immune system plays a critical role in Alzheimer's disease, and in particular, the innate immune system—which is the evolutionarily older part of the immune system, and the part that responds first to infections—plays an important role in Alzheimer's disease. However, this was not evaluated.
- *Microbiome:* Bacteria and other microbes living in the gut, mouth, nose, and sinuses, collectively called the microbiome, were not even mentioned.
- *Blood-brain barrier:* Often abnormal in Alzheimer's disease, it was not evaluated or even mentioned.

- *Body mass index:* A known risk factor for Alzheimer's disease and brain health in general, it was not noted. (This patient had a BMI of 33, considered overweight and far above what is optimal for cognition.)
- *Prediabetes:* Another driver of Alzheimer's, it was not even mentioned.
- *Volumetrics:* Although the MRI was utilized to exclude structural abnormalities, a critical test that measures the volumes of various brain regions was not included. This is a simple and very important addition to the MRI. Knowing which regions, if any, are shrinking can help identify whether Alzheimer's is present, which subtype is most likely, and whether the prognosis is better or worse. For example, generalized atrophy is more typical for type 3 (toxic) Alzheimer's disease, whereas atrophy confined to the hippocampus is more typical for types 1 and 2.
- *Targeted treatment:* Medication was prescribed without even knowing whether the patient did indeed have Alzheimer's disease.

For the evaluation and treatment of cognitive decline, the current state of affairs is truly a sad one:

- Patients often do not seek medical care because they have been told there is nothing that can be done. They fear the loss of their driver's license, the stigma of a diagnosis, and, in the US, the inability to obtain long-term care insurance.
- Primary care providers often do not refer patients to memory clinics, since they have been taught that there is no truly effective therapy. Therefore, they typically simply start donepezil (Aricept), often without a firm diagnosis.
- Specialists often put the patients through hours of

stressful neuropsychological testing, expensive imaging, and repeated spinal taps, and then have little or nothing to offer therapeutically.

We can do much better. We *must* do much better if we are to reverse the cognitive decline of Alzheimer's disease, MCI, and SCI. In this chapter you will find the metabolic evaluation that will pinpoint which factors are driving your cognitive decline, be it SCI, MCI, or any stage of Alzheimer's disease.*

Homocysteine

High levels of homocysteine are important contributors to Alzheimer's disease.† Remember how Alzheimer's disease results when the synapse-making signals in the brain are outweighed by the synapse-remodelling/destroying ones? Of the three causes of synapse loss—inflammation, loss of synapse-supporting (trophic) factors, and toxins—homocysteine is a marker of both the first and the second. It is a marker of inflammation, but it is also increased when nutritional support is suboptimal.

Homocysteine comes from eating foods with the amino acid methionine such as nuts, beef, lamb, cheese, turkey, pork, fish, shellfish, soy, eggs, dairy, or beans.

The methionine is converted into homocysteine, which in turn is converted back to methionine or cysteine, also an amino acid. That conversion requires vitamin B_{12}, vitamin B_6, folate, and the amino acid betaine. If you have healthy levels of these molecules

---

* Although the vast majority of cases of cognitive decline are the result of a neurodegenerative process, a small minority will have a different cause, such as a brain tumour. Prior to obtaining the metabolic evaluation recommended here, therefore, ask your doctor to exclude this possibility with an MRI or CAT scan.
† Also cardiovascular disease, stroke, and even some cancers.

you will have no trouble cycling your homocysteine, and its levels will remain healthily low. But if, like many people, you don't, your homocysteine will build up, damaging your blood vessels and brain. Any level above 6 micromoles per litre (also called micromolar) may pose a risk, and the higher the homocysteine, the greater the risk.[1] Although some of us can withstand chronically high homocysteine levels without developing Alzheimer's disease, they're a potentially important contributor to cognitive decline and, in particular, shrinkage of the hippocampus. In fact, the further your homocysteine increases above 6, the more rapidly your hippocampus atrophies.

TERI'S FATHER HAD DEVELOPED DEMENTIA AND ULTIMATELY had an autopsy showing classic Alzheimer's disease. Sharp and successful her entire life, Teri, 65 when she came to me, was an accomplished distance runner and writer, but when she turned 60 she began to note problems with focus and memory. Given her family history and symptoms, she underwent genetic testing, learning she was ApoE4-positive. When a laboratory blood test showed that her homocysteine was 16, she began the ReCODE protocol, and within three months noted improvement. But after six months her homocysteine had dropped only to 11, and her GP had said, "There is nothing I can do to reduce it further." It turned out that she had been taking cyanocobalamin (vitamin B_{12}) rather than methylcobalamin (methyl-B_{12}), folate rather than methyltetrahydrofolate, and pyridoxine rather than pyridoxal-5-phosphate. When she switched over to these three more active forms, her homocysteine dropped to 7. She has now been on the protocol for four years, remains mentally sharp and active, and recently had an amyloid PET scan that was normal, despite a single fleck suggestive of a small amount of amyloid.

GOAL: homocysteine < 7 micromolar.

Vitamins B_6, B_{12}, and Folate

Keeping your homocysteine optimally low requires sufficient levels of vitamins B_6, B_9 (folate), and B_{12}, all in their active forms. Pyridoxal-5-phosphate (P5P) is the active form of vitamin B_6, methylcobalamin is an active form of vitamin B_{12}, and methylfolate is an active form of vitamin B_9. When you get your blood tested for vitamin B_{12}, you'll see that the "normal" values are between 200 and 900 picograms per millilitre (pg/ml). This represents one of many examples in which doctors accept as "within normal limits" values that are clearly suboptimal.

For vitamin B_{12}, you'll often see a footnote to the results, explaining that "normal" levels between 200 and 350 may be associated with vitamin B_{12}-deficiency-related disease such as anemia and dementia! You therefore don't want to walk around with a "normal" B_{12} level of 300; you want a level over 500.

Many doctors order the MMA (methylmalonic acid) test instead of D_{12} itself, since as B_{12} declines, MMA increases. High MMA can therefore mean low B_{12}, and can be even more sensitive than B_{12}. The MMA test is fine as a complementary test to B_{12}, but since the MMA results can be quite variable, it is best to use it *with* and not instead of the B_{12} test.

For folate, the "normal" range is 2–20 nanograms per milliliter, but again, you don't want to be at the low end of normal. Aim for 10–25.

For vitamin B_6, you don't want to be at the low end (30–50 nanomoles per litre) *or* over the top, either (>110 nmol/L), since high levels can be toxic to a subset of your peripheral nerves, specifically the nerves that carry the sensations of touch and pressure, and are critical for gauging where your arms and legs are in space. You want to shoot for 60–100, taking P5P to get there; we'll talk about how much of each of these to take in the next section.

GOAL: vitamin B_{12} = 500–1500 pg/ml; folate = 10–25 ng/ml; vitamin B_6 = 60–100 mcg/L.

Insulin Resistance

High insulin and high glucose are two of the most important risk factors for Alzheimer's disease. As you may already have heard from any of a number of excellent books written on the subject, sugar is an addictive poison! The ATF—the US Bureau of Alcohol, Tobacco, Firearms and Explosives—might appropriately consider becoming the ATFS and adding sugar to its list of controlled substances, given the widespread damage wrought by high sugar intake. The human body is not designed to process more than about 15 grams per day of sugars, far less than in one soft drink (which has 40 to 100 grams, depending on the size of the soft drink), but our diets are laced with them, from sugary fizzy drinks to sweets to sweetened cereals and yoghurts—even shop-bought bread.

When you eat foods with a high glycaemic index—not just sugars but also starchy foods like white bread, white rice, white potatoes, and baked goods, among others—your body pours out large amounts of insulin in an attempt to keep glucose levels in check, because the glucose itself is toxic at high levels. That harms your cells in several ways. For one thing, the cells become insensitive to the constant flood of insulin just as commuters become insensitive to blaring car horns: when something is ever-present, you stop responding to it. This insulin resistance contributes not only to type 2 diabetes, fatty liver, and metabolic syndrome, but also to Alzheimer's disease. The reason: Insulin signalling is one of the most important signals for the support of neuron survival. Insulin binds to the insulin receptor and triggers signalling that supports neuronal survival; this survival signal is blunted by chronically high insulin levels. But that's not the only connection between chronically high insulin levels and Alzheimer's. The body degrades insulin after it does its job, using—among other enzymes—one called IDE (insulin-degrading enzyme). But IDE also degrades amyloid-beta, and if IDE is tied up degrading insulin, it isn't degrading amyloid-beta. Amyloid-beta levels therefore increase, contributing to Alzheimer's disease.

High levels of glucose cause problems beyond chronically high insulin levels. Glucose attaches to many different proteins, like remoras to a shark, interfering with their functioning. Hemoglobin A1c is a simple measure of one of many such altered molecules. These hitchhiking glucose molecules undergo biochemical reactions to produce advanced glycation end products, or AGE. These molecules wreak havoc by several different mechanisms. (1) Since the proteins with the AGE look different to your immune system, you may develop antibodies against your own proteins, triggering inflammation. (2) The AGE bind to their own receptor, called RAGE (receptor for advanced glycation end products), which also triggers inflammation. (3) The AGE cause free radicals to form, and these unstable reactive molecules damage anything they bump into, such as DNA and your cell membranes. (4) The altered proteins damage blood vessels, thus reducing nutritional support to the brain (contributing to type 2) and causing leakiness of the barrier between blood and brain (contributing to type 1).

For all of these reasons, it is crucial to know your glucose and insulin status. Your fasting insulin level should be 4.5 or below. Your fasting glucose should be 90 or lower, and your hemogloblin A1c should be less than 5.6 per cent.

KATRINA, A 66-YEAR-OLD WOMAN, DEVELOPED MEMORY problems, and felt a loss of sharpness in her mental ability. She repeatedly lost her car in parking lots, failed to recognize people she had met previously, and often lost her train of thought, making work difficult. She also had word-finding difficulty. Her laboratory evaluation revealed multiple metabolic abnormalities, including a high fasting glucose of 121 mg/dL indicating prediabetes, hemoglobin A1c of 5.6 per cent, fasting insulin of 4.2, and morning cortisol of 24.3 (indicative of stress, and contributing to high glucose levels). She began the ReCODE protocol, and four months later all of her symptoms had resolved, with concomitant improvement in her metabolic status, including a fasting glucose of 108 (still not optimal, but clearly improved), hemoglobin A1c of 5.5 per cent, fasting insulin of 3.4, and morning cortisol of 21.

GOAL: fasting insulin ≤ 4.5 microIU/ml; hemoglobin A1c < 5.6 per cent; fasting glucose = 70–90 mg/dL.

Inflammation, Inflammaging, and Alzheimer's Disease

There is a direct mechanistic link between inflammation and Alzheimer's disease. If you've ever called the police, then you have depended on them to distinguish the "good guys" from the "bad guys," capture the latter, and then return to the station. Imagine, however, that the police never leave your neighbourhood—that you lived in a police state, with ongoing shooting, damage, and death, and indiscriminant injury to both good and bad guys. This is just what is happening to most of us: our immune system—our internal police force—never stands down completely, and the resulting chronic (albeit mild) inflammation leads to cardiovascular disease, cancer, arthritis, accelerated aging—and Alzheimer's disease. The evidence that inflammation contributes to Alzheimer's disease is overwhelming. Besides being overactive in general, the chronically activated immune system sometimes attacks the body's own tissues.

Many assailants can call out this internal police force:

infections such as viruses, bacteria, or fungi; free radicals; advanced glycation end products; trauma such as bruises, sprains, and broken bones; damaged proteins or lipids such as oxidized LDL (low-density lipoprotein); and many other damaging agents. The internal police force response is remarkable, usually highly effective (which is why you are alive right now!), and complicated, with multiple branches.

There are several key measures of inflammation:

1. *C-reactive protein:* CRP is produced by the liver in response to any type of inflammation. Specifically, you want to know your hs-CRP (high-sensitivity CRP), since the standard CRP test is often too insensitive to distinguish optimal from mildly abnormal. Your hs-CRP should be below 0.9 mg/dL. If it is higher, you want to determine the source of the inflammation. This may be from too much sugar and other simple carbohydrates, or bad fats (for example, trans fats), a leaky gut (more on this later), gluten sensitivity, poor oral hygiene, specific toxins, or any of many other sources. When the source is located, it should be removed, and the hs-CRP rechecked.

2. *The ratio of albumin to globulin in your blood (A/G ratio):* This is a complementary measure of inflammation, and is best when it is at least 1.8.

3. *The ratio of omega-6 to omega-3 in your red blood cells:* While both of these fatty acids are important for health, omega-6s are pro-inflammatory while omega-3s are anti-inflammatory. The ratio of omega-6 to omega-3 should be less than 3 but not below 0.5, which increases risk of hemorrhage.

4. *Interleukin-6 (IL-6) and tumour necrosis factor alpha (TNFα):* Your internal police force uses a number of dispatchers to coordinate its response, and these are called cy-

tokines. Two of the many cytokines that may be increased in inflammatory (type 1) Alzheimer's disease are IL-6 and TNFα.

GOAL: hs-CRP < 0.9 mg/dL; albumin ≥ 4.5 g/dL; A/G ratio ≥ 1.8.
OPTIONAL TARGETS: omega-6:omega-3 ratio = 0.5–3.0; IL-6 < 3 pg/ml; TNFα < 6.0 pg/ml.

Vitamin D$_3$

Reduced vitamin D activity is associated with cognitive decline. Vitamin D travels through your blood and tissues like a Wi-Fi signal, entering your cells. Once inside, it binds to a receptor molecule called, appropriately enough, the vitamin D receptor (VDR), allowing the vitamin D to enter the nucleus (which houses your DNA) and turn on over 900 genes. Some affect bone metabolism, others suppress tumour formation, others reduce inflammation, and—crucially for the ReCODE protocol—others are essential for creating and maintaining brain synapses. These genes, and the vitamin D that activates them, are therefore crucial for keeping up the synapse-supporting side of the creation/destruction balance. When vitamin D is suboptimal, the right genes aren't correctly activated.

We get vitamin D when sunlight converts a cholesterol molecule, 7-dehydrocholesterol, into an inactive form of vitamin D, which is then converted into the active form.

Doctors used to think that a serum level of 25-hydroxycholecalciferol (an inactive form, it is the most commonly measured) of 20–30 ng/ml was healthy. I recommend aiming for 50 to 80. You can use the 100x rule to figure out your optimal dose of vitamin D (typically taken as vitamin D$_3$): subtract your current value (say, 20) from your goal (perhaps 50), and multiply that difference (30) by 100 to get the dose (3000) in IUs.

GOAL: vitamin D_3 (measured as 25-hydroxycholecalciferol) = 50–80 ng/ml.

Hormonal Status—Controversial but Critical

The word *hormone* comes from the Greek *horman*, meaning "to impel or set in motion." These signalling molecules are produced in one place, such as the pituitary, and then travel via the bloodstream to another site, such as the adrenal glands. Many hormones contribute crucially to optimal cognitive function, in particular by supporting synapse formation and maintenance, and when their levels drop, cognition declines as the synapses-eliminating side of that balance becomes dominant.

Thyroid status

Optimal thyroid function is crucial for optimal cognition, and suboptimal thyroid function is common in Alzheimer's disease. Thyroid hormone function is like the accelerator in your car—the more you push on it, the faster all of your cells go, metabolically speaking. You can measure the speed of your metabolism simply by taking your basal body temperature. Take a standard thermometer, shake it down, and place it next to your bed before you go to sleep for the night. Before getting out of bed in the morning, place the thermometer in your armpit for 10 minutes. It should read between 97.8 degrees and 98.2 degrees Fahrenheit. If it is lower, you likely have low thyroid function.

Your cellular metabolic speed also affects your reflexes. When your thyroid function is low, your reflexes will be slow. These can be measured by a machine called a Thyroflex, which is available in some doctors' offices in the US. It accurately records the speed of your brachioradialis reflex (the one that flexes your arm). If your thyroid is not functioning the way it should, then this—and all of your reflexes—will be slow.

Since thyroid function affects metabolic speed, it affects your heart rate and your mental sharpness. It can also have an impact on how long you sleep, whether you feel cold or hot, whether you gain weight easily, whether you become depressed, and many other health parameters. Furthermore, most people with dementia, mild cognitive impairment, and subjective cognitive impairment have suboptimal thyroid function. Therefore, it is essential to know your thyroid hormone status, which can be assessed by measuring levels of free T3 (this is the active T3), free T4, reverse T3, and TSH (thyroid-stimulating hormone).

Why so many? Most doctors check only TSH, but using this test alone fails to identify many patients who have suboptimal thyroid function.

TSH is produced by your pituitary gland in response to the command by TRH (thyrotropin-releasing hormone), which is made in the hypothalamus of your brain. When thyroid function declines, in theory TSH should increase to drive the thyroid gland to produce more thyroid hormone. Thus high TSH can indicate low thyroid function. "Normal" levels of TSH are considered to be 0.4–4.2 microIU/l, but anything over 2.0 is concerning.

In practice, however, you can have suboptimal thyroid function with a normal TSH. That's why I advise getting additional thyroid hormones checked:

Free T3: This is the active but short-lived thyroid hormone, molecules of which disappear after only one day (more keep being made, of course). Optimal levels are 3.2 to 4.2, measured in picograms per millilitre (pg/ml).

Free T4 is essentially the storage hormone, lasting about a week. Optimal levels are 1.3 to 1.8.

Reverse T3 inhibits thyroid activation. That is why one of the most important measurements of thyroid function is the ratio of free T3 to reverse T3. Levels of reverse T3 increase with stress and reduce the effectiveness of T3. The free T3:reverse T3 ratio should be at least 20.

OPTIMAL: TSH < 2.0 microIU/ml; free T3 = 3.2–4.2 pg/ml; reverse T3 < 20 ng/dL; free T3 x 100:reverse T3 > 20; free T4 = 1.3–1.8 ng/dL.

Oestrogens and progesterone

The role of oestrogens—oestradiol, oestriol, and oestrone—and progesterone in cognitive function remains controversial. But there is strong evidence for such a role. As noted above, oestrogen binds to its receptor and activates the enzyme (called alpha secretase or ADAM10) that cleaves APP so that it sends out the synapse-supporting duo of sAPPα and αCTF. Thus oestrogen is a crucial player in the prevention of dementia. Studies from the Mayo Clinic have shown that women who have their ovaries removed by age 40 (sometimes because they have a genetic risk of ovarian cancer) without hormone replacement therapy have double the risk of Alzheimer's disease.[2] Not only are oestrogens and progesterone important, so is the ratio of oestradiol to progesterone, since a high ratio is associated with "brain fog" and poor memory.

DIANE, A 55-YEAR-OLD LAWYER, HAD SUFFERED PROgressively severe memory loss for four years. On multiple occasions, she accidentally left the hob on when she left her home, forgot meetings, and scheduled multiple meetings at the same time because she didn't remember booking a previous one. Because she remembered almost nothing for more than a few minutes, she would record conversations and take copious notes on her iPad (unfortunately, she then forgot the password to unlock it). Her effort to learn Spanish as part of her job ended in failure. She became unable to perform her job. She often asked her children if they had brought home various household items that she had asked for, only to have them tell her she hadn't asked. She frequently became lost in midsentence, and was slow coming up with responses even in everyday conversations. One of her children said, "I went away to college, and when I came home, the person who was my mother was gone."

When Diane came to me, her homocysteine was 9.8, CRP normal at 0.16, vitamin D pretty good at 46, hemoglobin A1c fine at 5.3, oestradiol normal at 275, progesterone low at 0.4 (and thus oestradiol:progesterone ratio much too high at 687.5), insulin fine at 2.7, free T3 fairly good at 3.02, free T4 fine at 1.32, and TSH borderline high at 2.04.

After five months on ReCODE, however, she began to notice improvements. By ten months, four months after she had optimized her oestradiol:progesterone ratio, she had a virtually complete recovery. She no longer needed her iPad for notes or to record conversations. She was able to work again, learned Spanish, and began to learn a new legal speciality. She no longer became lost in midsentence, nor imagined that she had asked her children to do something she had not.

GOAL: oestradiol level = 50–250 pg/ml; progesterone = 1–20 ng/ml; oestradiol:progesterone ratio = 10:100 (and optimize to symptoms).

Testosterone

The sex steroid hormone testosterone, which is present in both females and males but at higher concentrations in males, supports the survival of neurons. Men in the lowest quintile of testosterone concentrations are at increased risk for Alzheimer's disease.

GOAL: total testosterone = 500–1000 ng/dL; free testosterone = 6.5–15 ng/dL.

Cortisol, pregnenolone, and dehydroepiandrosterone (DHEA)

Stress, which seems to be everywhere in our hyperconnected, über-productive, constantly competitive world, is one of the most important contributors to cognitive decline. Short periods of stress that you get over are less of a problem than the chronic unresolved stress that so many of us experience.

Stress activates the HPA axis—the hypothalamic-pituitary-adrenal axis—that I mentioned earlier. Our brain's hypothalamus produces corticotropin-releasing factor (CRF), which stimulates the pituitary gland to release ACTH (adrenocorticotropic hormone) into the blood. ACTH, in turn, causes the adrenal glands atop our kidneys to release cortisol and other stress-related hormones. High levels of cortisol damage neurons, especially in the hippocampus, making chronic stress an important contributor to hippocampal damage and thereby cognitive—and especially memory—decline.

Chronic stress can lead to dysfunction of the HPA axis (this was once called adrenal fatigue, but in fact the whole axis is out of whack). When this happens, the adrenal glands do not produce enough stress hormones to deal with stresses such as infections, toxins, or lack of sleep. You therefore become very sensitive to these stressors, which can exacerbate cognitive decline. Furthermore, a rapid reduction in cortisol can itself lead to the loss of neurons in the hippocampus.

Pregnenolone is the master steroid hormone from which all others—both sex steroids such as oestradiol and testosterone, and stress hormones such as cortisol and dehydroepiandrosterone (DHEA)—are derived. In periods of high stress, the pregnenolone is "siphoned off" to produce the stress hormones, leaving too little to produce the optimal levels of sex hormones. This "pregnenolone steal" is a common condition resulting in low levels of both pregnenolone and the sex steroids. It's why our interest in sex plummets when we are under great stress. Pregnenolone supports memory and is neuroprotective; thus an insufficient level of pregnenolone is a risk factor for cognitive decline.

DHEA, like pregnenolone, is a "neurosteroid" that supports response to stress, and it is usually measured as DHEA sulfate. For cortisol, pregnenolone, and DHEA sulfate, these can be measured simply in the blood serum or saliva, and if abnormalities are discovered, follow-up tests can be done by collecting urine over 24 hours. However, the blood evaluations are in most cases enough to determine whether there are suboptimal levels for cognition.

GOAL: cortisol (morning) = 10–18 mcg/dL; pregnenolone = 50–100 ng/dL; DHEA sulfate = 350–430 mcg/dL in women, and 400–500 mcg/dL in men.

Metal Detection—Not Just for Airports

Vulcan and Atlas—the copper:zinc ratio

Too much copper and too little zinc are associated with dementia. Professor George Brewer from the University of Michigan has spent his career studying the effects of copper and zinc on cognitive function, discovering that most of us are deficient in zinc but have excess copper. This is an especially prevalent problem in developed countries, possibly because of copper piping and in some cases from copper in vitamins, combined with zinc-poor diets and poor zinc absorption (often due to our stomachs producing less acid, especially as we age or take proton pump inhibitors for gastric reflux). More important, as Professor. Brewer has pointed out, aging is associated with lower zinc levels, and Alzheimer's disease with still lower zinc levels. Furthermore, patients with the toxic subtype of Alzheimer's disease (type 3) often have very low zinc levels—typically half those of healthy people—

and these low zinc levels cause them to be more sensitive to toxins such as mercury and the mycotoxins from mould. Moreover, zinc supplements enhance cognition,[3] as Professor Brewer found.

Because copper and zinc are competitive in a number of ways—for example, each inhibits the uptake of the other from the intestines—too much copper leaves us with too little zinc. Both are crucial to health, so you don't want too little of either. Although they are both metals, however, they are different in a crucial way: zinc is like Atlas, the strong and stable Greek Titan, whereas copper is like Vulcan, the god of fire. This is because the zinc ion (Zn^{++}) has a filled 3d atomic orbital—in other words, zinc is complete with electrons and is "full and happy"—whereas copper ions possess an incomplete 3d orbital and thus are unsatisfied. Therefore copper readily shuttles electrons in and out of the many proteins that contain it, and thus is a source of free radicals (molecules with unpaired electrons, which are typically damaging to our bodies and brains). On the other hand, zinc, as part of over 300 different proteins, does not have the ability to shuttle electrons the way copper does; therefore zinc does not produce free radicals the way copper does and is thus suitable for a strong, stable, structural role.

It has been estimated that as many as two billion people—more than a quarter of the world's population—are deficient in zinc. Zinc deficiency is especially prevalent in the elderly, with consequences that mirror Alzheimer's disease. For example, because zinc is critical for insulin synthesis, storage, and release,[4] zinc deficiency reduces insulin signalling, a critical feature of Alzheimer's. Zinc deficiency also increases the level of autoantibodies, a source of inflammation; increases oxidative damage and aging; reduces hormonal signalling and neurotransmitter signalling; and enhances sensitivity to toxins—all of which are characteristic of Alzheimer's or contribute to cognitive loss even in the absence of frank disease.

Your blood levels of both copper and zinc should be about 100 mcg/dL (micrograms per decilitre), and thus the ratio 1:1. Ratios of 1.4 or higher have been associated with dementia. Similarly, although most of your copper is bound by proteins such as ceruloplasmin, it is helpful to determine your free copper (the copper not bound by proteins), and you can easily calculate this by checking your copper, then subtracting three times your ceruloplasmin. For example, if your copper is 120 and your ceruloplasmin is 25, then your free copper is approximately 120 minus 75 = 45, which is too high—it should be less than 30.

Measuring zinc in red blood cells produces a more accurate reading than measuring it in serum, so you can also check your red blood cell zinc, which should be 12 to 14 mg/L.

GOAL: copper:zinc ratio = 0.8–1.2. Zinc = 90–110 mcg/dL (or red blood cell zinc = 12–14 mg/L).

ADDITIONAL, OPTIONAL TARGET: copper minus 3x ceruloplasmin ≤ 30.

Red blood cell magnesium and Ayurveda

Magnesium is critical for brain function. If you have Alzheimer's disease, which typically wreaks its worst and earliest havoc on the hippocampi and neighbouring entorhinal cortex, there is a good chance these memory-consolidating structures (one hippocampus on the left side of the brain and one on the right) are low in magnesium. Furthermore, achieving the level of magnesium that is optimal for brain cell function, Dr. Guosong Liu of MIT (now at Tsinghua University) showed, typically requires adding magnesium to the diet. In a clinical trial, Liu and his colleagues found that when magnesium is delivered to the brain by pairing it with a derivative of the amino acid threonine, cognition improves.[5]

When Guosong visited me at UCLA, we mused about the

irony of the approaches we each had taken. Here was Guosong, who had grown up in China, developing a targeted molecular monotherapy—a very Western tactic. And here I was, having grown up in the United States, developing a multipronged programmatic protocol that would be right at home in traditional Chinese medicine or Ayurvedic medicine.

As with zinc, measuring levels of magnesium in your red blood cells, where most of it resides, produces a more accurate reading than measuring it in serum. This is called RBC (red blood cell) magnesium. It should be between 5.2 and 6.5 mg/dL.

GOAL: RBC magnesium = 5.2–6.5 mg/dL.

Selenium, the firefighter (and glutathione, the water)

In the pantheon of metals, selenium is the firefighter. It works with the peptide glutathione (the firefighter's water) to mop up free radicals, the molecules with unpaired electrons that damage cell membranes, DNA, proteins, and overall cell structure and function. In protecting and restoring cellular health this way, glutathione is itself being used up and so must be constantly regenerated, just as firefighters need a constant supply of water. Low levels of glutathione can contribute to inflammation, toxicity, and loss of support for synapses—and, therefore to all three subtypes of Alzheimer's disease. Selenium plays a key role in regenerating glutathione when it is used up scavenging free radicals, so it is not surprising that reductions in selenium have been shown to be associated with cognitive decline.[6]

CAROL, 59, HAD BEEN SUFFERING FROM DECLINING MEMory and concentration for four years when she was evaluated at a major medical centre. Dementia runs in her family, and she carries one ApoE4 and one ApoE3, giving her an elevated risk of

Alzheimer's. A neuropsychological examination two years before suggested she had amnestic mild cognitive impairment, a common harbinger of Alzheimer's disease. Her cognition continued to decline, and an MRI showed marked atrophy of her hippocampus. It had shrunk so much that it was smaller than 99 per cent of hippocampi of people her age. That is a dire sign for someone with Alzheimer's symptoms.

Her evaluation identified mycotoxins in her urine, including one that was over 20-fold higher than the upper limit of normal. Since mycotoxins are often sensitive to glutathione, she was treated with intravenous (IV) glutathione plus the standard ReCODE protocol. Each time she received IV glutathione, her cognition improved for the remainder of the day, but slipped back by the next morning. However, over the next several months, her husband and her doctor noted clear and sustained improvements in her cognition. Her MoCA (Montreal Cognitive Assessment) score increased from 14 (average for full-blown Alzheimer's is 16.2) to 21 (not yet normal, which is 26–30, but markedly improved, and now much better than the average Alzheimer's patient).

GOAL: serum selenium = 110–150 ng/ml; glutathione (GSH) = 5.0–5.5 micromolar.

Heavy metals and the Mad Hatter

Heavy metals like mercury are neurotoxic, and most of us do not know we have been exposed to them. Remember the Mad Hatter from *Alice in Wonderland*? His character has a historical basis. From the eighteenth to well into the twentieth century, hat makers used a form of mercury to remove fur from rabbits and other small animals, and in the felt-making process, the mercury was released into the air. Their "madness," including memory loss, depression, insomnia, tremors, irritability, and extreme social phobia, was actually mercury poisoning. Although few of us make felt hats these days, let alone use mercury to do so, we are nevertheless exposed to this heavy metal and its compounds when we eat fish with high levels of it. (The larger the fish and the longer it lives, the more mercury it typically has, so tuna, swordfish, orange roughy, and shark are of particular concern, whereas the "SMASH fish"—salmon, mackerel, anchovies, sardines, and herring—are safer.) This type is organic mercury, typically methylmercury—mercury bound to a methyl group (one carbon and three hydrogen atoms), which occurs when microorganisms act on the mercury. The other major source of mercury is dental amalgams, the old-fashioned fillings so many of us have or had. This is inorganic mercury. Methylmercury and inorganic mercury can be distinguished in blood and urine tests, so you will know whether the mercury in your system is mostly from fillings or fish.

Mercury can induce the signature pathology of Alzheimer's disease—amyloid-beta plaques and neurofibrillary tangles. As if that weren't enough, methylmercury also destroys the parts of glutathione that mop up free radicals.

Arsenic, lead, and cadmium can also affect brain function. Although arsenic became infamous as the favourite poison of little old ladies, a more common source of exposure is groundwater, especially in the western United States, Taiwan, and some areas of China. Arsenic is also present in chicken, but is much lower in organic chicken. Chronic exposure to high levels of arsenic has been associated with impaired executive function (including problem solving, planning, organizational ability, and other forms of higher-order thinking), reduced mental acuity, and deterioration of verbal skills, as well as depression[7]—exactly the sort of deficits that occur with type 3 (toxic) Alzheimer's disease. Arsenic also affects the hypothalamic-pituitary-adrenal axis, which is often involved in type 3 Alzheimer's. One practical note for checking your arsenic—it is best to avoid seafood for at least three days before having your blood drawn for an arsenic level, since seafood often contains some nontoxic organic arsenic compounds, which give a false-positive reading.

Scientists have known for decades that lead impairs cognitive function, leading to lower IQs in exposed children. Exposure to lead—typically through old paint and dust in cities—also increases amyloid formation later in life, rodent studies have shown.[8] In people, there is both epidemiological and toxicological evidence that lead raises the risk of age-related cognitive decline.[9]

Cadmium is better known as a carcinogen than a dementogen, but rodent studies have suggested that it acts with lead and arsenic to enhance Alzheimer's-type changes in the brain.[10] You can be exposed to cadmium from cigarette smoking or working in chemical factories. Cadmium is also used in paints, especially brilliant yellows and reds—Monet used cadmium yellow for his garden paintings—but fortunately, current paints are engineered chemically so that the cadmium is much less available for toxicity.

There are several ways to check your mercury level, but most are relatively insensitive. Mercury is often measured in your blood, but since mercury sits in deposits in bone, brain, and other tissues, the blood level is not a very sensitive indicator. You can have mercury toxicity without high levels in your blood. Collecting urine is a more sensitive indicator. The standard has been to collect urine, typically over six hours, following the administration of a chelating agent, that is, a chemical that grabs onto the mercury tightly and pulls it out of the tissues. A very sensitive test called the Mercury Tri-Test, developed by Quicksilver Scientific, measures mercury from hair, urine, and blood without the need for chelation. It will tell you not only whether you have a toxic level of mercury but also whether it is organic (from fish) or inorganic (from dental amalgams). Quicksilver also offers a very sensitive blood test for other metals, including calcium, chromium, copper, lithium, magnesium, molybdenum, selenium, zinc, aluminium, antimony, arsenic, barium, cadmium, cobalt, lead, mercury, silver, strontium, and titanium.

While we are on the subject of metals, can aluminium cause Alzheimer's disease? No one knows. This was a common claim years ago, but follow-up studies have not supported it. On the other hand, it has not been completely disproven either.

GOAL: mercury, lead, arsenic, and cadmium all < 50th percentile (by Quicksilver); or, if blood levels are evaluated by a standard laboratory: mercury < 5 mcg/L; lead < 2 mcg/dL; arsenic < 7 mcg/L; cadmium < 2.5 mcg/L.

Sleepiphany: Sleep and Sleep Apnea

Sleep apnea is extremely common, usually goes undiagnosed, and contributes to cognitive decline. The Greek god of sleep is Hypnos, son of Nyx (the night) and Erebus (the darkness), and father to the gods of dream. Sleep is one of the most powerful weapons in the large anti-Alzheimer's armamentarium. Yet in our hypercompetitive society, it is a badge of honour to pull all-nighters or get by on only a few hours of sleep per night.

Sleep affects cognition through multiple fundamental mechanisms:

1. It alters the cellular anatomy of your brain, allowing a cleansing. The space in between brain cells, called the extracellular space, expands during sleep, allowing more calcium and magnesium ions to flow through. Like the tide scouring a shoreline, this is thought to flush out cellular debris, including amyloid.
2. Sleep is also associated with a reduced formation of the amyloid.
3. We don't eat when we're asleep. Fasting improves our insulin sensitivity.

4. During sleep, our brain cells activate autophagy, the process of "self-eating" that recycles cellular components like damaged mitochondria and misfolded proteins, improving cellular health. Without autophagy, your cells would collect dysfunctional components—it would be like powering all of your devices with worn-out batteries. Your cells need nice fresh batteries and shiny new parts, so you need sleep.
5. Sleep is also a time of repair. Growth hormone increases during sleep, repairing cells, and new supportive brain cells are produced during sleep, among the many reparative processes that occur during sleep.

No wonder sleep deprivation impairs cognition. Moreover, it increases the risk of obesity, diabetes, and cardiovascular disease, all risk factors for Alzheimer's disease. It gives us cravings for the sugar, unhealthy fats, and other unhealthy foods that give us an Alzheimer's-inducing metabolic profile.

Even if you try to get a solid seven or eight hours of shut-eye each night, if you have sleep apnea, in which your breathing periodically stops, jolting you semi-awake, you are not getting the quality sleep you need for cellular restoration. That makes sleep apnea an important contributor to cognitive decline. Yet an estimated 75 per cent of patients with sleep apnea are never diagnosed, partly because that used to require an expensive overnight stay at a hospital sleep centre. Fortunately, it is now possible to test for sleep apnea at home for a relatively modest sum, and there are wearable devices that can detect sleep apnea. Those of us who are most at risk for sleep apnea, and who should therefore be evaluated for it, include people who snore, males who are middle-aged or older, people who are overweight, people with short, thick necks, and those who are chronically tired during the day. Ideally, however, anyone experiencing cognitive decline would be evaluated, since sleep apnea (as well as other sleep disorders) is a readily addressable contributor. The evaluation will yield an AHI (apnea-hypopnea index), which is the number of times per hour you have stopped or nearly stopped breathing. Some people may have an AHI of 100, but normal is fewer than 5 and the target is 0.

Beyond sleep apnea, if you find that you are negative for sleep apnea but still fall asleep frequently during the day, ask your doctor about UARS—upper airway resistance syndrome—since it can mimic sleep apnea yet is not detected by sleep apnea studies. Your practitioner may refer you for a different test for UARS, such as a sleep study with oesophageal pressure monitor or a sensitive pulse oximetry study.

GOAL: AHI (apnea-hypopnea index) of fewer than 5 events per hour (preferably 0).

Cholesterol and Other Lipids

We all worry about having high cholesterol. Testing for cholesterol became popular in the 1950s and 1960s, along with other crazes like the Twist, the Hula-Hoop, fins on automobiles, and bell-bottoms. Somehow, though, when those other fads went the way of puka shell necklaces, the cholesterol craze kept the vitality of Dick Clark. (For you youngsters, Dick Clark was the *American Bandstand* host who kept his youthful looks well into his old age, and was thus called America's Oldest Teenager.) We still want to know our cholesterol level! But here's the real Twist: the Hula-Hoop has a lot more to offer (it is, after all, an excellent way to exercise) than measuring your cholesterol. This is because many people with "high cholesterol" have no problem with vascular disease, and many with "normal cholesterol" have significant vascular disease. Vascular disease itself is a contributor to cognitive decline, because it raises the risk of Alzheimer's disease and can cause vascular dementia, which is typically associated with many small strokes.

Perhaps surprisingly, *low* rather than high cholesterol is associated with cognitive decline. When total cholesterol falls below 150, you are more likely to suffer brain atrophy—shrinking. Cholesterol is a key part of cell membranes, including those of brain cells. What you *don't* want is *damaged* cholesterol and its related lipid particles—these are the bad guys. So measuring total cholesterol to assess cardiovascular risk is like counting people in each home to estimate how many criminals there are: of course some homes will have many people but no criminals, and other homes will have only a few inhabitants, of whom most are criminals. We want to measure the criminals directly, not guess from the total number of people: measure the oxidized LDL, small dense LDL, or LDL particle number, along with the degree of inflammation (oxidized LDL and hs-CRP that was described earlier).

GOAL: LDL-p (LDL particle number) = 700–1000; OR sdLDL (small dense LDL) < 20 mg/dL or < 20% of LDL; OR oxidized LDL < 60 U/l; total cholesterol > 150 (yes, *more than* 150, not less than).

Vitamin E

Vitamin E is an important protector of your cell membranes, an antioxidant with an anti-Alzheimer's effect. What we call "vitamin E" is actually a set of compounds, with names like tocopherols and tocotrienols, that interact with the fatty cell membranes, protecting them from damage by scavenging free radicals. It is one of the very few molecules that has been shown in a clinical trial, as a monotherapy, to slow cognitive decline, albeit modestly, in Alzheimer's disease.[11] Although there are multiple tocopherols and tocotrienols in vitamin E, you can get a pretty good idea of your status by having a laboratory test for alpha-tocopherol.

GOAL: vitamin E (measured as alpha-tocopherol) = 12–20 mcg/ml.

Vitamin B₁ (Thiamine)

Thiamine—vitamin B$_1$—is critical for memory formation. Thiamine deficiency is associated with alcohol abuse and malnutrition-associated memory loss, called Wernicke-Korsakoff syndrome. Thiamine levels can also drop if you eat foods that contain thiamine-degrading enzymes, such as tea, coffee, alcohol, and raw fish (although this is an uncommon cause of serious vitamin B$_1$ deficiency). Whether thiamine plays a role in the cognitive decline associated with Alzheimer's disease or aging is less clear; nevertheless, it is important to know if your levels of thiamine are sufficient to support healthy cognition. This is best done by measuring thiamine pyrophosphate (TPP) in your red blood cells.

GOAL: serum thiamine = 20–30 nmol/l OR red blood cell thiamine pyrophosphate (TPP) = 100–150 ng/ml of packed cells.

Gastrointestinal Permeability ("Leaky Gut")

It has been only a few years since leaky gut was recognized as a medical problem, and it has turned out to be a very common one, contributing to inflammation and other conditions. Most of us go to great lengths to ensure that our homes are safely sealed, preventing burglary, animal entry (have you ever walked in to find a stray cat eating the cat food? Or found a snake coiled in your house?), water leaks, and other unwanted intrusions. It is similarly crucial to maintain tight barriers in your body, starting with your gut.

Ideally, the cells that line your gastrointestinal tract maintain tight junctions (a protein complex with occludin acts as the caulk between the cells). These tight junctions keep food on the correct side—inside your gut. Molecules resulting from digestion, like the amino acids into which proteins are broken down, are then transported into gut lining cells and from there into the bloodstream, which carries these nutrients to cells throughout the body.

But imagine that the GI tract is leaky, as can occur due to gluten sensitivity, damaging chemicals like those in pesticides, soft drinks or alcohol, sugar, processed foods, and preservatives; inflammation, chronic stress, yeast, and medications such as aspirin or acetaminophen. Now it is not just amino acids, the simplest sugar molecules, like glucose or fructose, and vitamins that reach the bloodstream. So do larger fragments. These fragments are recognized by the immune system as foreign, triggering inflammation. Since inflammation is a key cause of Alzheimer's—especially type 1—it is crucial to keep these large protein fragments from leaking out of the gut and into the bloodstream.

Another reason to keep things sealed tight: Gut porosity allows other invaders such as bacteria and yeast, and fragments thereof, to enter your bloodstream. Again your immune system responds, sometimes in a way that causes collateral damage to your own tissues because, to the immune cells, they resemble the invaders. The result is autoimmune conditions in which you have persistent low-level inflammation and, in the worst case scenario, autoimmune diseases such as multiple sclerosis, rheumatoid arthritis, or lupus erythematosus. The chronic inflammation can also contribute to Alzheimer's disease.

VICKY, 16 YEARS OLD, HAD ALWAYS BEEN VERY HEALTHY, when she developed repeated rashes, arthralgias (painful joints), and swollen knuckles, exacerbated by cold weather. She gained weight, missed her periods repeatedly, and had difficulty focusing on conversations and schoolwork. She was evaluated by two different internationally recognized experts in rheumatology and underwent biopsy of the rash on her hands. It showed that she had vasculitis—inflammation of the blood vessels. She tested positive for lupus and was told that she was at high risk for the development of chronic severe lupus and that there was no current treatment.

Vicki sought evaluation by an integrative physician, who found that she had leaky gut, multiple food sensitivities including to gluten and dairy, reduced thyroid function, reduced oestradiol, and insulin resistance. After she spent several months on a programme of dietary restriction, gut healing, and hormonal balancing, all of her symptoms remitted: the rashes disappeared, she returned to her normal weight, her oestradiol level normalized, her menses returned, and her mental focus improved. Follow-up testing for lupus was negative. Every time Vicki reintroduced small amounts of gluten to her diet, however, she again developed arthralgias. Vicki continues to be healthy, without any evidence of lupus, nine years after her symptoms began.

What does a case of a young woman with leaky gut developing vasculitis, arthritis, and reduced hormonal function—due to the autoimmunity triggered by a leaky gut—have to do with Alzheimer's disease? Everything. One of the most important contributors to Alzheimer's disease is inflammation, and one of the most common ways to create systemic inflammation is a leaky gut.

Thus it is critical to know your gut permeability. There are several ways to do this. One is through a test in which you ingest two different sugars, lactulose and mannitol: mannitol passes through the gut barrier normally, whereas lactulose doesn't—unless the gut is leaky. After entering the bloodstream, one or both of these sugars will appear in the urine. The mannitol in the urine tells you that the gut is not failing to absorb, but if there is also lactulose, it indicates a leaky gut. Alternatively, you can evaluate the immunological response that occurs when the gut is breached by fragments that shouldn't pass through. The body produces antibodies against bacteria that enter the bloodstream via the leaky gut, resulting in antibodies to the LPS (lipopolysaccharide) on the bacteria's surface. Similarly, antibodies to the barrier protein, zonulin/occludin, indicate leaky gut. These can be measured in an antibody array called Cyrex Array 2. Since food sensitivities can cause a leaky gut, it is helpful to test for those, either through Cyrex Arrays 3 and 4, or by eliminating suspects from your diet, then reintroducing them one at a time and seeing if symptoms such as joint pains or bloating or abdominal pain occur.

GOAL: Cyrex Array 2 (or other measure of gut permeability) negative.

Blood-Brain Barrier Permeability

A growing list of disease-causing bacteria, viruses, fungi, and other microbes have turned up in the brains of patients with Alzheimer's disease. Wait, what? Don't microbes in your brain indicate meningitis or encephalitis? It's not quite that simple. Meningitis and encephalitis are active infections with inflammation, like a hot war. The presence of low levels of pathogens is more like a cold war, a slow wearing down and suboptimal functioning. There is something of a standoff, with neither side waging all-out war.

For a disease like Alzheimer's that was not thought to be infectious, finding pathogens in the brain is both surprising and concerning. A bacterium called *Porphyromonas gingivalis* (*P. gingivalis*) has turned up repeatedly in Alzheimer's brains, as have some of the proteins made by this microbe.[12] Where does it come from? Your mouth! Other oral bacteria, too, have been found, including *Fusobacterium nucleatum* and *Prevotella intermedia*. So has the *Herpes simplex* virus (HSV), which lives for years in the nerve cells that supply your face and lips—your trigeminal ganglion cells—and sallies forth during times of stress or sunburn to cause cold sores. It can also migrate right back up the same nerve and into the brain, producing the mild, chronic inflammatory response—the cold war kind—associated with Alzheimer's disease.

Do you remember syphilis? Many of us have forgotten this disease, which was an important cause of dementia before it became easily diagnosed by lab test and effectively treated with penicillin. Syphilis is caused by *Treponema pallidum*, a type of bacterium called a spirochete because of its corkscrew shape. *Treponema* can live in the body for decades, eventually infecting the brain and causing dementia years after the initial infection. In some ways, Alzheimer's is the neurosyphilis of the twenty-first century, since it involves a chronic inflammatory response of the brain. However, whereas syphilis is caused by a single organism, in Alzheimer's disease inflammation may be caused by many different organisms or even by so-called sterile inflammation—not from invading pathogens but from causes such as poor diet.

The Lyme disease spirochete, *Borrelia burgdorferi,* has also been found in the brains of Alzheimer's patients. Carried by the tiny deer tick *Ixodes*—which lives all over the eastern and western United States, Europe, middle-latitude Asia, and into northern Africa—*Borrelia* gets into your body when deer ticks attach to you, bite, and inject saliva that includes the spirochete. Just over half of patients who develop Lyme disease are also infected with additional microbes carried by the ticks, including *Ehrlichia* (which infect white blood cells), *Babesia* (a relative of the malaria parasite, which infects red blood cells), and *Bartonella* (which infect blood vessels). The brains of many patients with Alzheimer's disease also harbour fungi.

The Alzheimer's brain, as you can see, is a veritable zoo of organisms. No single one is the cause of the disease, the way *Borrelia* is the cause of Lyme disease and *Treponema* is the cause of syphilis. Instead, Alzheimer's actually reflects a protective response to many different infectious, inflammatory, or toxic insults.

How do these organisms get into the brain? Normally the brain is protected by the blood-brain barrier, but this barrier can break down. Just as you can develop leaky gut, you can develop a leaky blood-brain barrier. Microbes can also access the brain through the nose (as cocaine users know eye-openingly well), through the gut (the vagus nerve that connects the gut to the brain stem), and even through the eye. Dementogens likely reach the brain via all of these routes. In Alzheimer's, there is evidence of abnormalities in the blood-brain barrier very early in the disease. Furthermore, multiple studies have found that the nasal and sinus access to the brain is also a critical determinant in Alzheimer's disease type 3.

For all these reasons, it is helpful to know the status of your blood-brain barrier. The Cyrex Array 20, which evaluates the response to leaked blood-brain barrier proteins, can assess that.

GOAL: Cyrex Array 20 negative.

Gluten Sensitivity and Related Sensitivities

The gut-brain connection is critical for cognition. Although only about 5 per cent of people develop coeliac disease, which is associated with severe gluten intolerance, the majority of us may suffer damage to our gastrointestinal tracts—and especially the tight junctions between the cells—from gluten. This is discussed at length by my friend and colleague Dr. David Perlmutter in his bestselling book *Grain Brain*. Since gluten sensitivity can cause leaky gut, which (as described earlier) can trigger the kind of chronic inflammation that leads to Alzheimer's, it is important to evaluate gluten sensitivity. One way is to assess tissue transglutaminase antibodies in serum, which is a standard blood test. Another is to undergo Cyrex Array 3 testing, which evaluates antibodies to different regions of the two molecules that make up gluten. Sensitivity to rye, barley, sesame, oats, or rice—which can also cause leaky gut—can be evaluated using the Cyrex Array 4.

> SLIM, 74, STARTING LOSING HIS MEMORY AT AGE 67. HE was evaluated at two of the nation's leading medical centres and told that he had probable Alzheimer's disease. Although his evaluation did not include genetic testing, an inflammatory evaluation, amyloid imaging, a PET scan, or MRI volumetrics, he began to receive mailings offering him participation in clinical trials for candidate drugs for Alzheimer's disease.
>
> After his memory and cognition kept declining, Slim was evaluated further. His MRI showed general cerebral atrophy, with hippocampal volume at only the 5th percentile for his age. His Cyrex Array 2 indicated a leaky gut. Array 20 was also positive, indicating a leaky blood-brain barrier. Array 5 disclosed autoantibodies: his immune system was reacting against his own proteins, including the brain proteins myelin basic protein and glutamic acid decarboxylase. After he spent a year on the ReCODE protocol, along with avoidance of gluten, testing indicated that he no longer had a leaky gut or a leaky blood-brain barrier, and his progressive cognitive decline had ceased.

GOAL: tissue transglutaminase antibodies negative OR Cyrex Array 3 negative and Cyrex Array 4 negative.

Autoantibodies

If your immune system is waging war on your own brain, as Slim's was, it is important to know that, since autoantibodies—especially those that attack brain proteins—are an important contributor to cognitive decline. The Cyrex Array 5 assesses a host of autoantibodies.

MINDY BEGAN TO EXPERIENCE DEPRESSION FOLLOWING A hysterectomy at age 50, despite hormone replacement therapy (which may or may not have been adequate). Four years later, she began to experience difficulty finding words, driving, and following recipes and other instructions. She felt disoriented and, after her son left home, increasingly depressed. Mindy's husband noted that her mood and cognition both improved markedly after she had several days of rest, but declined markedly with sleep deprivation, viral illness, or other stressors. Her MoCA (Montreal Cognitive Assessment) was 19 (normal is 26–30), indicating significant impairment compatible with Alzheimer's disease. A neuropsychological evaluation found she could not remember her own family history (which, relatives said, did not include dementia), exhibited paucity of speech, had poor semantic fluency, confabulated (made up answers to mask forgetting) on memory tests, and was unable to smell. All of the symptoms pointed to deficits in her brain's frontal, temporal, and parietal lobes. Her MRI was deemed normal, but quantitative volumetrics were not performed. Her PET was abnormal, with reduced glucose utilization in the parietotemporal and frontal regions, characteristic of Alzheimer's disease.

Testing revealed levels of an autoantibody against her thyroid protein (thyroglobulin) more than 2,000 times normal. She also had high C4a and TGF-β1, which are characteristic of the activation of the innate immune system and typical for type 3 Alzheimer's disease. Her ApoE genotype was 3/3. Mindy was treated for CIRS (chronic inflammatory response syndrome, which can be induced by mycotoxins or Lyme disease or other pathogens), with cholestyramine (this binds toxins in the gut) and intranasal VIP (vasoactive intestinal peptide, which supports neurons), along with the ReCODE protocol. Over the next several months, she improved markedly: she was able to read and remember once again, able to follow directions, able to navigate, and overall, able to function much better.

GOAL: Cyrex Array 5 negative.

Toxins, Type 3 Alzheimer's Disease, and CIRS

Surprisingly, toxins are turning out to be an important cause of Alzheimer's disease. The toxicology course I took in medical school did not prepare me to understand the sea of toxins we swim in every day. We inhale poisons, we ingest toxins, we absorb toxins through our skin, we produce endogenous toxins as biochemical reaction by-products, we are exposed to toxic electromagnetic fields and radiation. Most of the time we don't sense these toxins, so we don't even have a chance to avoid them. But there is growing evidence that many of them are the "dementogens" I mentioned earlier.

Several years ago, when my colleagues and I first discovered that there is a balance between the cellular signalling associated with synapse formation and maintenance vs. synapse reorganization and remodelling, we set up a way to test any chemical for its effect on this critical balance. In other words, we would screen for both dementogens and their opposites, compounds that boost synapse formation and maintenance. We screened through every FDA-approved drug, as well as other chemicals that were potential drugs, looking both for potentially valuable candidates that would shift the balance in the positive direction—toward more memory formation and maintenance—and potential dementogens that shifted the balance in the negative direction. Surprisingly, several of the statins, the widely prescribed cholesterol-lowering drugs, seemed to tip the balance in the wrong direction: they caused the kind of APP cleavage that produces one of the "destructive quartet" that induces cell death.[13] Interestingly, the statin that did this most powerfully, cerivastatin (previously sold as Baycol), had been taken off the market in 2001 after it was linked to more than fifty deaths worldwide and to side effects such as the death of muscle cells.

Another set of dementogens, found repeatedly in type 3 Alzheimer's patients, is mycotoxins,[14] made by moulds such as *Stachybotrys*, *Aspergillus*, *Penicillium*, and *Chaetomium*. What? Alzheimer's disease due to mould? Sadly, there is more and more evidence that moulds contribute to some cases, likely at least 500,000 patients in the United States alone. Therefore, it is good to check your mycotoxin exposure, as I'll describe below, if you or any family members have experienced cognitive decline.

Over the past two decades, Dr. Ritchie Shoemaker has studied the effects of mycotoxins in thousands of patients, as he recounts in his 2010 book, *Surviving Mold: Life in the Era of Dangerous Buildings*. Dr. Shoemaker described a syndrome that he named CIRS—chronic inflammatory response syndrome. The symptoms are many and varied—including asthma, chronic fatigue, fibromyalgia (widespread muscle, tissue, and bone pain and tenderness), nosebleeds, rashes, shortness of breath, cognitive decline, headaches—and all appear to be related to the chronic activation of the ancient part of the immune system, the so-called innate immune system.

Here's how it works. Imagine that a bomb goes off in a building in your town. There will be an immediate emergency response, prior to any specifics about the perpetrators, including mobilizing emergency services, curfews, and text alerts to stay indoors until more information is available. Then, when surveillance cameras identify the perpetrators, the response can focus on those responsible for the blast. This is exactly how your innate immune system works. It sends out all-purpose infection-fighting cells and signals. Only later does another part of the immune system, called the adaptive immune system, produce antibodies that specifically target and destroy the microbes causing the infection. Normally, once the infection is vanquished, both immune responses stand down.

But what would happen if the surveillance cameras never identified the perpetrators? The curfew and the general high level alert would remain in place. That's what happens with CIRS. The innate system is activated by mycotoxins or other invaders, often for years, but the adaptive system does not recognize and destroy them. What determines whether our surveillance cameras are working? Genetics. For 75 per cent of us, the cameras are on, so we are in good shape. But for the other 25 per cent, the cameras are off for mycotoxins (or for some other microbial invaders such as the Lyme disease *Borrelia*). That leaves the innate immune system chronically activated, producing the constant inflammation that sets the brain down the path to Alzheimer's. Fortunately, we can find out easily whether we are in the 75 per cent or the 25 per cent, using a genetic blood test for HLA-DR/DQ. Furthermore, we can find out if our innate immune system is activated using simple blood tests for C4a, TGF-β1, and MSH. In addition, we can undergo urine testing for the presence of the most dangerous mycotoxins: trichothecenes, ochratoxin A, aflatoxin, and gliotoxin.

GOAL: C4a < 2830 ng/ml; TGF-β1 < 2380 pg/ml; MSH = 35–81 pg/ml; HLA-DR/DQ with no CIRS propensity; urinary mycotoxin test negative for trichothecenes, ochratoxin A, aflatoxin, and gliotoxin derivative.

Mitochondrial Function

Like tiny batteries, mitochondria supply the energy that allows our cells to function. They convert the energy locked in your food and the oxygen you breathe into the molecule ATP, which in turn powers your cells. The name *mitochondria* comes from the Greek for "little granular thread," and these amazing batteries are actually the descendants of bacteria that invaded our cells over a billion years ago, taking up long-term residence much to our own advantage.

Since many chemicals damage mitochondria, it is helpful to know whether you have been exposed to these, especially in significant amounts or over a long period of time. The list includes antibiotics (which kill bacteria, and thus can be toxic to our mitochondria since they are descendants of bacteria), statins, alcohol, L-DOPA (prescribed to treat Parkinson's disease), griseofulvin (prescribed for fungal infections), acetaminophen (paracetamol), NSAIDs (aspirin, ibuprofen, and related drugs), cocaine, methamphetamine, or AZT (azidothymidine, used for viral infections including HIV/AIDS). In addition, ApoE4 may be associated with mitochondrial damage.

There is not a simple blood test that assesses mitochondrial function, although there are some indirect tests, such as testing organic acids. Mitochondrial testing currently available is directed more at discovering mitochondrial defects in childhood diseases than in cognitive decline, so improved methods of testing are sorely needed. Until they arrive, the best way to test for the alterations in mitochondrial function that may occur with cognitive decline are with breath tests, nuclear magnetic resonance tests, mitochondrial DNA sequencing, and muscle biopsies. For now, with respect to the identification of potential contributors to cognitive decline, it is helpful to know whether there has been exposure to the mitochondrial-damaging agents listed above.

GOAL: no exposure to mitochondria-damaging agents.

BMI (Body Mass Index)

An unhealthy body mass index (BMI) raises your risk for cognitive decline. You can find simple online calculators or do it yourself. Simply multiply your weight (in pounds) by 703, divide by your height in inches, then divide that by your height again. Here's an example: if you are 5 feet 6 inches tall (66 inches) and weigh 130 pounds, then your BMI = 130 x 703, or 91,390; divided by your height of 66 inches gives 1,384; divided by 66 again gives 20.98, which you can round to 21. This is very good: for optimal cognition, BMI should be between 18 and 25. BMIs over 26, and especially above 30, increase the risk of type 2 diabetes, which in turn increases the risk of Alzheimer's disease. Less is known about the risk of BMIs below 18, but these may be associated with suboptimal nutrition and hormonal status, so the goal is to keep the BMI between 18 and 25.

BMI is not the optimal indicator for metabolic status, however. Visceral fat status, which you can determine with imaging techniques such as ultrasound or an MRI, is a more accurate indicator, especially the presence of fat in the liver. You can determine this with a body composition analyzer, and you want to have a Tanita score of 1–12. Another good indicator of metabolic status is your waistline: it should be less than 35 inches for females or 40 inches for males.

GOAL: BMI (body mass index) = 18–25; waistline < 35 inches (women) or < 40 inches (men).

Genetics

Genetics affect your risk for Alzheimer's disease, but your Alzheimer's fate is by no means written in your DNA. Instead, much more than you might expect, you are in control of your own fate. In order to optimize your control, you want to know your genetic status: for one thing, your optimal diet will be different if you are ApoE4 positive than if you are ApoE4 negative.

Many of us are leery about genetic testing. It can be scary to find out about one's own DNA. However, keep in mind that genetic testing can be empowering, as in the ApoE/diet example above. You can have your entire genome sequenced, which costs about $1,600 £1,200. You can sequence your exome (the part of the genome that codes for proteins) for about $600 £460. You can simply find out how many copies of ApoE4 you have (0, 1, or 2).

Or you can undergo testing at a company like 23andMe, which assesses a large number of SNPs (single nucleotide polymorphisms, which are variations within your genes). As I write this, however, 23andMe has stopped offering interpretations of health-related genes including ApoE (they still report things like genes for eye colour). You therefore need to request your own file, which will be emailed as a zip file, then have it analyzed by a website service like Promethease or MTHFR Support. Also, about 15 per cent of the time, 23andMe testing fails to determine the ApoE status. And 23andMe doesn't test for all of the disease-causing variants in every gene related to Alzheimer's.

Postscript: In April 2017, the FDA approved ten DNA tests from 23andMe, including one for late-onset Alzheimer's disease risk, which evaluates ApoE status.

GOAL: Knowing your ApoE status.

OPTIONAL TARGET: Knowing your status on all SNPs related to neurodegeneration, such as APP, PS1, PS2, CD33, TREM2, CR1, and NLRP1.

Quantitative Neuropsychological Testing

It is critical to know where you stand with your memory and other aspects of cognition, such as organizing, calculating, and speaking. There are many ways to do this. The simplest is to take the MoCA (Montreal Cognitive Assessment) test, which is freely available online and takes only about ten minutes (http://dementia.ie/images/uploads/site-images/MoCA-Test-English_7_1.pdf). There are three versions, so you can repeat it without concern that any improvement comes from having seen the same test before. A normal MoCA score is 26 to 30; 19 to 25 is associated with MCI; 19–22, if accompanied by difficulties with activities of daily living, usually means that MCI has converted to dementia, whether from Alzheimer's disease or another cause; and scores lower than 19 indicate dementia.

There are other simple tests, such as the Mini-Mental State Examination (MMSE) or SAGE (Self-Administered Gerocognitive Examination), but they are less sensitive to early changes than the MoCA, and thus more useful for more severely affected patients. Although these tests, including MoCA, assess multiple cognitive functions and thus brain regions, more extensive tests, also available online, are more sensitive to early changes and also provide more detailed analysis of brain function. These include CNS Vital Signs, BrainHQ, Dakim, Lumosity, and Cogstate, all of which calculate your percentile (that is, that you are above X per cent of the people your age) for multiple areas of function.

Neuropsychologists can conduct more extensive evaluations, providing sensitive, in-depth assessment of multiple domains of cognitive function. But these evaluations can take several hours and be stressful, and therefore some people elect to avoid the potentially harmful stress and instead use a shorter test, such as those described above.

GOAL: Obtain baseline cognitive performance as percentile for age or as MoCA score (out of a perfect 30).

OPTIONAL TARGET: Complete standard neuropsychological testing and obtain percentile scores for multiple cognitive domains.

Imaging, Cerebrospinal Fluid, and Electrophysiology

What does your brain look like? Imaging the brain can show which, if any, regions, have shrunk and which are using less energy—and therefore are less active—than they should be. MRI with volumetrics provides raw data that programmes like Neuroreader and NeuroQuant use to assess percentile scores—again, that the volume of your hippocampus, say, is above X per cent of that of people your age. Neuroreader, for instance, calculates that for 39 brain regions. Anyone who has symptoms of cognitive decline, no matter how early, should obtain an MRI with volumetrics. And anyone at high risk—for example, based on a strong family history or genetics—should consider it. For those who are asymptomatic and not at high risk, this is optional.

PET (positron-emission tomography) scans are often helpful when the diagnosis is in question, such as when it is otherwise difficult to distinguish between frontotemporal dementia and Alzheimer's disease. In the latter, the FDG-PET shows a characteristic pattern of reduced glucose metabolism in the temporal and parietal regions, often including the posterior cingulate and precuneus, which are often impaired in Alzheimer's.

Amyloid PET scans show amyloid accumulation in the brain. But because amyloid accumulation may occur without Alzheimer's disease, and conversely, Alzheimer-pattern cognitive decline may occur without amyloid, it is not yet clear whether this approach will be helpful in diagnosis. In fact, ongoing studies aim to determine just that. If you happen to find that you have a positive amyloid PET scan in the absence of symptoms, it suggests that you should be serious about prevention. However, the pattern of amyloid accumulation does not correlate well with the region of brain displaying symptoms: that is, as an example there may be amyloid in the frontal lobes, which are responsible for behaviour, executive function, and many other functions, but the patient's main symptom may be memory loss that is related to temporal lobe dysfunction. In contrast, a newer type of PET scan—tau PET scans—tend to show abnormalities that correlate more closely with symptoms.

Cerebrospinal fluid (CSF, from a spinal tap) is also optional, but again helpful if the diagnosis is in question. In Alzheimer's disease, there is a characteristic reduction in the amyloid-beta 42 in the CSF and an increase in total tau and phospho-tau.

EEG (electroencephalography), another optional test, can be very helpful in determining whether there is any evidence of seizure activity. Although seizures occur in only about 5 per cent of people with Alzheimer's disease, the EEG may reveal unsuspected seizure activity even though there is no twitching or other outward signs of seizures (so-called nonconvulsive seizures). If that is the case, then anticonvulsants (antiseizure medications) can be prescribed.

GOAL: brain MRI with volumetrics normal, showing no areas of atrophy.

OPTIONAL TARGETS: negative FDG-PET scan, negative amyloid PET scan, negative tau PET scan, and/or normal EEG, without seizure activity or slowing.

Novel and Soon-to-Appear Tests Critical for Cognitive Decline Assessment

1. Neural exosomes

The most exciting new area of testing for Alzheimer's disease, Alzheimer's disease risk, and response to therapeutics involves neural exosomes, tiny fragments of cells and materials expelled from cells. This could be a neurological Holy Grail: a simple way to evaluate brain chemistry and neuronal signalling by taking a blood sample. How can this be? How can we learn about brain signalling by analyzing blood? Well, picture yourself as a private investigator, and you want to know what is going on inside an impregnable mansion. You can't get in, but you need to know what is going on. So what do you do? You go through the household rubbish, right?

It turns out that the brain—the nearly impregnable mansion inside your skull—puts out neural exosomes, detritus and secretions from cells that enter your bloodstream. These tiny fragments of cells and materials are quite small, averaging about one-seventieth the width of a red blood cell. There are lots of these exosomes in your blood—billions in each ounce of blood! So this is really cool: you take a small blood sample, isolate the neural exosomes, and determine many critical parameters of brain biochemistry, exactly what you need to know to determine where you stand with risk for cognitive decline, whether you have type 1 or 2 or 3 Alzheimer's, and most important, whether the treatment programme is working or needs to be tweaked.

Professor Edward Goetzl and his colleagues at the University of California, San Francisco, and the National Institutes of Health have found the signature of Alzheimer's disease in neural exosomes, including increases in amyloid-beta and phosphorylated tau.

They've also found the signature of insulin resistance in the neural exosomes of patients with Alzheimer's disease, discovering that it can occur up to a decade prior to the diagnosis of Alzheimer's. These findings are, in all likelihood, just the tip of the exosomal iceberg, since this approach has the potential to assess neurotransmitter pathways, hormonal signalling, trophic factor signalling, vitamin effects on neural function, trauma effects, vascular compromise, therapeutic responses, and many more biochemical signatures in the brain. You can see why I am so enthusiastic about this approach.

I sit on the scientific advisory board of a new company, NanoSomiX, that works with Professor Goetzl and evaluates neural exosomes. When this test becomes available, it will be helpful to know your neural exosome level of amyloid-beta 42 (the main one associated with Alzheimer's), phospho-tau, cathepsin D (a protease that is increased in exosomes from patients with Alzheimer's disease), REST (which indicates levels of trophic support), and phosphorylation ratio of IRS-1 (indicating insulin resistance or sensitivity).

GOAL: normal neural exosome levels of amyloid-beta 42, phospho-tau, cathepsin D, REST, and phosphorylation ratio of IRS-1.

2. Retinal imaging

Another exciting new approach to early evaluation and assessment of risk for cognitive decline is retinal imaging. Although you can image amyloid in the brain with an amyloid PET scan, this detects only relatively large collections of amyloid. It does not reveal whether the amyloid is in the blood vessels or not, and does not lend itself to looking at relatively rapid changes in single amyloid plaques.

The back of the eye, or retina, is an extension of the brain and therefore reflects what is ongoing in there. That makes evaluating the retina for amyloid plaques a highly promising approach. It is possible to identify many, often hundreds, of very small plaques, map the location of each, and then follow up after treatment to see whether the number of plaques has declined. At several hundred dollars instead of a few thousand, retinal imaging is much less expensive than amyloid PET scans of the brain. It also identifies much smaller plaques, which may be more accurate sentinels of treatment effects, and also has the potential to reveal whether the amyloid affects the retina's blood vessels (and by extension, likely the brain's as well) in addition to the neurons and synapses themselves. This is important because amyloid in blood vessels can, in rare cases, lead to hemorrhage (bleeding), and thus in such cases blood-thinning agents such as fish oil and aspirin must be assiduously avoided.

NeuroVision Imaging, cofounded in 2010 by neurosurgeon Dr. Keith Black of Cedars-Sinai Medical Center and entrepreneur Steven Verdooner, provides retinal imaging and imaging equipment. As I write, the company is conducting clinical trials of whether this approach can detect early Alzheimer's disease and track response to treatment.

GOAL: retinal imaging negative (/normal range) for amyloid plaques.

3. Neurotrack and the mesial temporal lobe (novel object recognition)

One of the most helpful tests in evaluating the loss of memory in lab rodents is the novel object recognition (NOR) test. Imagine that you awoke tomorrow morning and were surprised to see a brand-new red sports car in your driveway. You would likely spend some time with it, looking, touching, sitting in it, specifically because of its newness and the novelty of finding something unexpected in your world. In comparison, familiar items like your old car would receive much less of your attention and time. However, if you had no memory, you would not be able to recognize the new car as new; everything would seem new. So it is with rodents. Those with good memories spend extra time with novel objects, whereas those with poor memories do not. Therefore, measuring novel object recognition is how many laboratories evaluate Alzheimer's-related brain changes in rodents and also test candidate therapies. For instance, research has shown that damage to the mesial temporal lobe deep in the brain impairs the ability to remember and recognize what's new in one's environment, and occurs early in Alzheimer's disease.

This same memory-based preference for novelty can be tracked in people. In 2016 Neurotrack released the Imprint Cognitive Assessment Test, a five-minute web-based visual cognitive assessment that, by tracking eye movements, detects which objects and other stimuli people recognize as novel. It thus detects impairment of the hippocampus and nearby structures, identifying people who have dysfunction of this region and may be manifesting the pathophysiology of Alzheimer's disease.

GOAL: normal preference for novel objects.

Other Considerations

Historical/lifestyle features

Critical as laboratory tests are for identifying genetic and biochemical factors that may be contributing to cognitive decline, life history can also provide crucial clues to what is causing it. It is therefore important to know if you currently or have ever:

- suffered head trauma. (Have you ever been knocked unconscious? Had an automobile accident? Played contact sports?)
- had general anaesthesia (and how many times). General anaesthesia combines some toxicity of the anaesthetics with what is often imperfect oxygenation, and this can affect brain function.
- have dental amalgams. These expose you to inorganic mercury.
- eat high-mercury fish. This exposes you to organic mercury.
- take certain medications (especially any with brain effects, such as benzodiazepines like Valium, antidepressants, blood pressure pills, statins, proton pump inhibitors, or antihistamines).
- used street drugs.
- drink alcohol (and how much).
- smoke cigarettes.
- practise good oral hygiene. Poor oral hygiene can contribute to inflammation.
- have surgical implants (artificial hips or breast implants, for instance).
- have liver, kidney, lung, or heart disease.
- snore. This may suggest the possibility of sleep apnea.
- consume hot-pressed oils (like palm oil). These hot-pressed oils lose some of their vitamin E during the heat processing and therefore may be damaging to your brain.
- eat foods high in trans fats or simple carbohydrates. These have multiple effects, such as vascular damage and insulin resistance.
- have chronic sinus problems. These may alert you to exposure to moulds and their related mycotoxins.

- have gastrointestinal problems such as bloating or recurrent diarrhoea. This may tip you off that you have a leaky gut.
- have mould in your house, car, or workplace. Most people do not realize that such exposure is a risk factor for cognitive decline.
- eat processed foods or nonorganic foods. These often contribute to insulin resistance and toxin exposure.
- had tick bites. Ticks carry over 70 different pathogens, such as the Lyme disease *Borrelia*, and the chronic inflammation associated with these may contribute to cognitive decline.
- take proton pump inhibitors for reflux. These reduce the stomach acid needed for digestion, and therefore reduce the uptake of zinc and vitamin B_{12}, among other nutrients.
- use makeup, hair spray, or antiperspirant. These relate to toxic exposure.
- don't sweat much (one important route for toxin elimination).
- been constipated (bowel movements also eliminate toxin).
- don't drink enough purified water (urine also removes toxins).

Any of these might be contributing to cognitive decline. When there are at least thirty-six possible holes in your roof—thirty-six factors that are causing synapse-destroying reactions to outweigh synapse-preserving or -creating ones—it is helpful to prioritize which to address first. Like the lab tests described above, your personal and medical history can help do that.

Finances

How expensive are all these tests? Depending on your health insurance or what is available through your GP and the NHS, it might be a great deal out of pocket or very little. For instance, many insurance policies in the US cover tests such as hemoglobin A1c, homocysteine, and CRP. In general, healthcare has focused more on reaction than prevention, but that is beginning to change, and therefore groups like Medicare may cover more tests in the future as their scientific and clinical value becomes more clearly established. In the UK, some but not all of these tests may be done under the NHS. Your out-of-pocket costs might therefore be a few hundred pounds to several thousands. However, considering the personal and family effects of cognitive decline, to say nothing of nursing home care for those with full-blown Alzheimer's, I firmly believe that preventing and addressing cognitive decline is an excellent investment. Hopefully, as more and more people who undergo such testing and follow the ReCODE protocol experience reversal of cognitive decline, insurers will begin to cover these critical tests.

Summary: The Cognoscopy

Let's summarize what you need for your cognoscopy, which I recommend for anyone 45 years or older. I realize it sounds daunting when you first read about the tests, but in fact the list is pretty straightforward: the combination of blood tests, genetic tests, simple online cognitive assessment, and MRI with an automatic computer assessment of brain volumes provides crucial clues to what is causing cognitive decline or putting you at risk for it. Basically, the elements of the cognoscopy reveal which synapse-destroying processes might be at work in your brain, and which synapse-maintaining ones might not be firing on all cylinders, leading to the synapse loss that causes the loss of memory and cognitive abilities. This is in stark contrast to the laborarory tests now done for cognitive decline, none of which actually pinpoints its underlying cause or causes.

Table 2. Summary of the key tests and optional tests for the ReCODE protocol.

	Critical tests	Target values	Optional tests	Comments
Genetics	ApoE	Negative for ApoE4	Whole genome, exome, or SNPs	Saliva or blood
Blood tests				
Inflammation vs. cellular protection	hs-CRP	<0.9	IL-6, TNFα	
	Homocysteine	<7		
	Vitamins B$_6$, B$_{12}$, and folate	60–100 (B$_6$) 500–1500 (B$_{12}$) 10–25 (folate)		
	Vitamins C, D, E	1.3–2.5 (C) 50–80 (D) 12–20 (E)		Vitamin D is measured as 25-hydroxy-cholecalciferol
	Omega-6: omega-3 ratio	0.5 to 3.0		
	A/G ratio (albumin: globulin ratio)	≥1.8 >4.5 (albumin)		
	Fasting insulin, glucose, hemoglobin A1c	≤4.5 (fasting insulin) 70–90 (fasting glucose) <5.6 (A1c)	Neural exosome studies (p-tau, Aβ42, REST, cathepsin D, and IRS-1 phos. ratio)	
	Body mass index (BMI)	18–25		
	LDL-p or sdLDL or oxidized LDL	700–1000 (p) <20 (sd) <60 (ox)		
	Cholesterol, HDL, triglycerides	>150 (cholesterol) >50 (HDL) <150 (TG)		
	Glutathione	5.0–5.5		

	Critical tests	Target values	Optional tests	Comments
	RBC thiamine pyrophosphate	100–150		
	Leaky gut, leaky blood-brain barrier, gluten sensitivity, autoantibodies	Negative		
Trophic support	Vitamin D	50–80		
	Oestradiol (E2), progesterone (P)	50–250 (E2) 1-20 (P)		
	Pregnenolone, cortisol, DHEA-sulfate	50–100 (preg) 10–18 (cort) 350–430 (DHEA, women) 400–500 (DHEA, men)		
	Testosterone, free testosterone	500–1000 6.5–15 (free)		
	Free T3, free T4, reverse T3, TSH	3.2–4.2 (fT3) 1.3–1.8 (fT4) <20 (rT3) <2.0 (TSH) fT3:rT3 >20		
Toxin-related	Mercury, lead, arsenic, cadmium	<5, <2, <7, <2.5, respectively	<50th percentile (Quicksilver)	
	Copper:zinc ratio	0.8–1.2	RBC zinc; ceruloplasmin	
	C4a, TGF-β1, MSH	<2830 (C4a) <2380 (TGF-β1) 35–81 (MSH)	MMP9, VEGF, leptin, VIP, ADH, osmolality	If abnormal, add MARCoNS culture and VCS testing
	HLA-DR/DQ	Benign HLA-DR/DQ		

	Critical tests	Target values	Optional tests	Comments
Metals (excluding the heavy metals listed as toxins)	RBC-magnesium	5.2–6.5		
	Copper, zinc	90–110 (both)		
	Selenium	110–150		
	Potassium	4.5–5.5		
	Calcium	8.5–10.5		
Cognitive performance	CNS Vital Signs, BrainHQ, or equivalent	>50th percentile for age, improving with practise	Novel object recognition	
Imaging	MRI with volumetrics	Hippocampal, cortical volume percentiles steady (or increasing) for age, >25th percentile	Retinal imaging	Neuroreader or NeuroQuant
Sleep	Sleep study	AHI < 5/hr.		
Microbiomes	Gut, oral, nasal	No pathogens		

CHAPTER 8

ReCODE: Reversing Cognitive Decline

Change will not come if we wait for some other person or some other time. We are the ones we've been waiting for. We are the change that we seek.
—BARACK OBAMA

AFTER YOU HAVE identified the biochemical, genetic, and other factors that are causing synaptic destruction to outweigh synaptic formation and maintenance, the ReCODE protocol calls for addressing each of these.

EDWARD WAS A BRILLIANT PROFESSIONAL WHO HAD BUSInesses on both the East and West Coasts. He would meet with his accountants and add columns of numbers immediately in his head, before the accountants could do so on their calculators. As he approached 60, however, he began to have memory problems. One day at the gym, he panicked when he forgot the combination to his locker, and his lock had to be cut. His memory continued to decline. He could no longer add columns of numbers rapidly in his head, and he had difficulty remembering people he had met. A PET scan revealed a pattern typical of Alzheimer's disease. Edward had extensive quantitative neuropsychological evaluations, which supported the PET results. He learned he was ApoE4-positive, providing further evidence that his developing dementia was due to Alzheimer's disease. He continued to decline, according to neuropsychological evaluations, at a rate that accelerated when he was 67, and two years later his neuropsychological evaluation revealed such marked memory loss and cognitive dysfunction that the neuropsychologist suggested he wind down his business and plan for the full-time care he would soon need.

His wife brought him to meet with me, and he began on the ReCODE protocol in December 2013. After six months his wife called me: "Edward has clearly improved, but that is not the most striking effect," she said. Rather than declining more and more rapidly, as he had for the eighteen months prior to starting the protocol, the first noticeable effect was that the decline ceased completely. A few months later, he began to improve.

His wife, his coworkers, and Edward himself all noticed a clear improvement. Instead of closing his business, he opened a third location. After Edward had been on the protocol for two years, I suggested that he undergo another neuropsychological evaluation. Since he had had one in 2003, 2007, and 2013, getting nothing but worse and worse news, he was reluctant. He pointed out that the neuropsychologist had always been pessimistic—it was Alzheimer's disease, after all, so the neuropsychologist was "hanging crepe," preparing Edward for the worst. Furthermore, the neuropsychologist did not believe that anything could be done: in thirty years of practice, he had never seen anyone in Edward's condition improve. There was another consideration. "I know I'm doing better, and my wife and coworkers know I am doing better," Edward said. "What if the neuropsychologist tells me that I'm wrong? That it's all wishful thinking?"

His concerns raised an important paradox, called the observer effect (a cousin of the Heisenberg uncertainty principle), in which the measurement of something (Edward's mental capacity) affects the very thing that is being measured (ditto). Was it truly in his best interest to undergo quantitative neuropsychological testing yet again? Why risk casting doubt on his apparent progress?

We discussed this, and Edward recognized that, if there truly was objective, quantitative evidence of improvement, given that he had well-documented Alzheimer's disease, his case could be helpful to many others. He agreed to take the examination, which was performed by the same examiner who performed those in 2003, 2007, and 2013. (Using the same examiner increases the accuracy and reliability of such longitudinal tests.) This occurred twenty-two months after Edward had started the ReCODE programme.

My wife and I were driving up the California coast, from Los Angeles to San Francisco, when my mobile phone rang. It was the neuropsychologist, asking me to come in to go over the testing results for Edward. In his thirty years of practice, he said, he had never seen such results: Edward's California Verbal Learning Test (CVLT), which assesses verbal memory abilities and is a test that is often markedly abnormal in Alzheimer's patients, had improved from the 3rd percentile to the 84th percentile. His auditory delayed memory had improved from the 13th percentile to the 79th. His reverse digit span had improved from the 24th percentile to the 74th. Other tests had improved as well. However, the neuropsychologist was most interested in Edward's processing speed, which had improved from the 93rd to the 98th percentile. I asked him why he had focused on this more modest improvement. The reason, he said, is that processing speed is a limiting feature in other, non-Alzheimer's processes such as traumatic brain injury and aging itself. Maybe the protocol Edward had used might help in those situations and others beyond Alzheimer's disease, he said.

As I write this, Edward has followed the ReCODE protocol for three years. He continues to work full-time. He opened that third office. He is asymptomatic. "I have allowed myself to think about the future once again when I talk to my grandchildren," he told me.

As I've mentioned, in people who already have symptoms of cognitive decline we almost always find between ten and twenty-five blood chemistry values that are suboptimal. In contrast, in people without such symptoms, we typically identify only three to five. (Please keep that in mind as you undergo testing: because your brain is resilient, it can function at pretty near its optimal level even if not every value is ideal.) The important point is that each of these values can be returned to a healthy, even optimal, value. Before I explain the specifics of how to do that, let me note the key conceptual points important for treatment:

1. *For each abnormality identified, we want to go beyond simply "normal" and get all the way to optimal.* This is because we need to do everything possible to correct the imbalance between synapse preservation and synapse destruction that is the root cause of cognitive decline and which, in its earliest stages, puts you at risk for such decline. As an example, a serum homocysteine level of 12 micromoles/litre is considered to be "within normal limits." But studies have clearly shown that it is suboptimal.[1] Similarly, a vitamin B_{12} level of 300 picograms per millilitre is "normal," but is often associated with symptoms of B_{12} deficiency. We want to get homocysteine to 6 µmol/L or lower, get B_{12} to 500 pg/mL or higher, and similarly optimize each value.

2. *We want to address as many of the abnormalities as possible, not just one.* The more of the thirty-six or so "holes" in the roof that we can patch, the better the chance of averting or reversing cognitive decline—much better than with any single therapy.

3. *For each treatment, the goal is to address the root cause of the problem it targets.* For example, if we find evidence of ongoing inflammation, we want to identify its cause and remove it, not simply suppress the inflammation while allowing its underlying cause to fester.

4. *The ReCODE programme is personalized, based on the laboratory values we find to be abnormal.* Because no two

people have the same lab values, a one-size-fits-all approach makes no sense.

5. *Just as for other chronic illnesses such as osteoporosis, cancer, and cardiovascular disease, there is a threshold effect.* Once enough of the network components have been optimized, the pathogenetic process can be halted or reversed. Therefore, even though most patients will not follow every step of the protocol, following enough steps to exceed the threshold—that is, to reach the tipping point from synapse destruction to synapse maintenance and preservation—should be sufficient.

6. *The programme is iterative.* You don't simply obtain a prescription and sit back assuming the problem is solved. The programme is broken down into phases, and you tweak it to optimize it for yourself, guided by the ongoing results.

7. *Drugs are the dessert, not the entrée.* The ReCODE protocol is a platform on which to add specific drugs. A single drug without the programme does not address the complexities of the process optimally, and therefore will not prevent or arrest—and certainly will not reverse—cognitive decline. Drugs can be a powerful part of the treatment arsenal, but they are not the first line of treatment, and for many people who start early, drugs may not even be necessary.

8. *The earlier you start treatment, the greater your chance for complete reversal.* When we think of cancer, we think of pain and wasting and, all too often, a relatively rapid death. In contrast, Alzheimer's is a sneaky, seductive reaper, and we go for years ignoring our minor slipups and "senior moments" before realizing only too late that yes, it really is Alzheimer's. Now that we have diagnostics to "see it coming" years ahead of significant symptoms and a programme to address the problem early on, the goal is to find out where

you stand as early as possible—preferably in the presymptomatic or subjective cognitive impairment period (which may last a decade or two), when there is known risk from family history, genetics (ApoE4, for example), or biochemistry (e.g., prediabetes). *What this really means is that virtually no one should have to die from Alzheimer's disease*, as long as the diagnosis is made early enough, the treatment programme is complete, adherence is good, and follow-up with continued optimization is regular.

9. *For just about every element of ReCODE, there is a workaround or crutch if you need it, so don't lose heart!* You can make it work. It might be helpful to have a health coach or adopt your protocol in phases, starting with the easiest steps. But please remember, whatever it takes is preferable to the progressive dementia characteristic of Alzheimer's disease.

Now that you know the basic concepts, let's go over the specifics of how to prevent and reverse cognitive decline. Since these instructions are personalized, some will depend on your laboratory values, whereas others will be helpful to everyone.

Homocysteine

If your homocysteine is over 6 micromoles per litre, you can lower it by taking vitamin B_6, B_{12}, and folate. In one study, homocysteine was normalized when patients took 20 milligrams of B_6, 0.5 milligrams of B_{12}, and 0.8 milligrams of folate. Since many of us have biochemistries that fail to turn the vitamins we ingest into their active forms, however, it's best to take the activated forms of these vitamins. Therefore, if your homocysteine is above 6, start by taking the pyridoxal-5-phosphate (P5P) form of vitamin B_6, 20 to 50 milligrams each day; the methylcobalamin (methyl-B_{12}) and adenosylcobalamin forms of B_{12},

1 milligram in total each day; and the methyltetrahydrofolate (methyl-folate) form of folate, starting with 0.8 milligrams (and as high as 5 milligrams) each day.

After three months, recheck your homocysteine to make sure that it has indeed dropped to 6 micromoles per litre or lower. In the uncommon cases in which it hasn't, simply add 500 milligrams daily of glycine betaine (also called trimethylglycine, available in capsule form). Recheck homocysteine in another three months. If it is still high, reduce the methionine (the amino acid from which the body makes homocysteine) in your diet by limiting consumption of foods such as nuts, beef, lamb, cheese, turkey, pork, fish, shellfish, soy, eggs, dairy,* and beans.

Insulin Resistance

If your fasting insulin is over 4.5 milli-international units per litre, your hemoglobin A1c over 5.5 per cent, or your fasting glucose over 93 milligrams per decilitre, you likely have insulin resistance, arguably the single most important metabolic contributor to Alzheimer's disease development and progression. As described above, many of us become insulin resistant from diets high in simple carbohydrates such as sugar, processed food full of high-fructose corn syrup, sedentary lifestyles, and stressful jobs and home lives. Fortunately, there are actually many ways to combat this insulin resistance. The solution is a very effective combination of DESS (diet, exercise, sleep, and stress reduction)—which is so important for your cognitive health that you might call them your "desstiny"—along with some simple supplements and, as a last resort, medication. Let's start with diet, a

---

* Whenever I mention dairy, I mean not only the products of cow's milk but also those from sheep's and goat's milk.

surprisingly powerful part of the overall programme to reverse cognitive decline.

Why is food so critical to brain function? As a teenager, I felt just fine after eating a cheeseburger and french fries—why not just continue eating what I feel like eating? Here's why. One of the most intriguing abilities of our bodies is to switch between modes that are optimal for a given activity—sleep and wakefulness, for example. Sleep is great for restoration and recharging, but wakefulness is much better for playing basketball. Similarly, there is a fundamental switch between the use of carbohydrates or fats as our main source of energy. Our ancestors typically burned fats when the hunt went well and meat was plentiful, whereas they burned carbohydrates when the fruit ripened in the autumn and when they gathered plants and tubers. The ability to switch back and forth is called metabolic flexibility. Now imagine you were trapped in a nether state in which you were neither asleep nor awake: you would not receive the full benefits of either state. You certainly would not do very well at basketball, but you also would not restore and recharge as well as if you had truly slept. That is what happens when your metabolic flexibility is compromised, something that turns out to be very common in those with insulin resistance—and thus most people with Alzheimer's disease. Your cells cannot optimally metabolize either carbohydrates or fats.

Restoring insulin sensitivity and metabolic flexibility are critical for trophic factor production, response to the trophic effects of insulin, minimizing inflammation, reducing obesity and lipid storage, improving cardiovascular status, optimizing hormones and hormonal responses, and thereby enhancing cognition. Therefore, cheeseburgers and fries are on the dementogen list; they should be on our plates rarely if at all. Below are the details of the optimal diet.

The Anti-Alzheimer's Diet: Ketoflex 12/3

None of us wants to eat a boring or bad-tasting diet! Fortunately, there are well-rounded, delicious menus that help prevent and reverse cognitive decline. I'll focus on the points most relevant to cognition. As you'll see, there is certainly more than one way to succeed—for example, you can follow these principles as a vegetarian or an omnivore and get the same benefits.

1. *The first part of Ketoflex 12/3 refers to ketosis,* the process in which your liver produces specific chemicals called ketone bodies (acetoacetate, beta-hydroxybutyrate, and acetone) by breaking down fat. This occurs when you are running low on carbohydrates, your body's first source of energy. Mild ketosis, it turns out, is optimal for cognitive function: beta-hydroxybutyrate increases production of the important neuron- and synapse-supporting molecule BDNF (brain-derived neurotrophic factor), among other effects.

To promote ketosis, you combine a low-carbohydrate diet (minimizing simple carbs such as sugars, bread, white potatoes, white rice, soft drinks, alcohol, candy, cakes, and processed foods), moderate exercise (at least 150 minutes per week of brisk walking or something more vigorous), and fasting for at least twelve hours between your last meal of the night and your first of the next morning (more on this in a minute). Consuming fats such as MCT oil (medium-chain triglyceride oil) or unsaturated fats such as olive oil or avocado or nuts also promote mild ketosis. This will switch your metabolism from carbohydrate-burning and insulin resistant, which promotes Alzheimer's disease, to fat-burning and insulin sensitive, which helps prevent it. Remember: As metabolism goes, so goes cognition.

When you shift from a predominantly carbohydrate-burning mode to a predominantly fat-burning one, you may have some carbohydrate craving or feel lethargic. If so, it helps to take MCT (medium-chain triglyceride) oil as capsules (containing 1 gram of MCT oil) or liquid (1 teaspoon). Alternatively, you can take coconut oil, which is a solid, anywhere from a teaspoon to a tablespoon three times per day. Too much coconut oil too quickly may cause diarrheoa, so it is best to start with a teaspoon and then work up to a tablespoon. Both MCT oil and coconut oil, along with the fasting, low-carbohydrate diet, and exercise, will help create mild ketosis. But both may also have drawbacks for ApoE4-positive individuals, as I'll discuss in greater detail below, so if you are ApoE4-positive, think of MCT and coconut oil as temporary crutches to ease your segue into fat-burning mode.

Since ketosis is a critical component of the overall programme, it is helpful to purchase a ketone meter, which measures the ketone beta-hydroxybutyrate in your blood. The meters cost about £27 (see Appendix B) and can be purchased online. (Ketones can also be measured in the urine, which is less accurate, or by a ketone breathalyzer test.) Aim for about 0.5 mM to 4 mM beta-hydroxybutyrate.

2. *The flex in Ketoflex 12/3 refers to a flexitarian diet.* This is a largely plant-based diet with an emphasis on vegetables, especially nonstarchy ones. It is best to include both uncooked vegetables, such as those in salads, and cooked ones, and to include as many colours as possible, from deep green to bright yellow and orange. Some fish, poultry, and meat are fine, but remember that meat is a condiment, not a main course. Ideally, you would limit your consumption of meat to 50 to 70 grams per day. One rule of thumb is to consume one gram of protein for each kilogram of your weight. For example, if you weigh 70 kilograms (154 pounds), you

should consume about 70 grams of protein. For comparison, 90 grams of fish includes about 20 grams of protein. What happens if we eat more than one gram of protein for each kilogram of our body weight? Biochemically, there is some conversion to carbohydrates, and this may contribute to the very insulin resistance we are trying to reverse. Furthermore, quantity is not the only important guideline, quality is also a consideration: the type of fish or meat is important, as I'll detail below.

3. *The 12/3 part of Ketoflex 12/3 refers to fasting times.* Fasting is a highly effective way to induce ketosis, improve insulin sensitivity, and thereby enhance cognition. The *12* refers to 12 hours between the end of dinner and the next day's first meal or snack. People with the ApoE4 genotype should aim for 14 to 16 hours, which may sound more draconian than it is: if you finish dinner at eight, you simply hold breakfast until at least ten A.M. The *3* refers to 3 hours as a minimum time between the end of dinner and bedtime, so if, for example, you typically go to bed at eleven P.M., then you should finish your evening meal no later than eight and avoid snacks after then. That will keep your insulin level from spiking before bedtime, something that can contribute not only to insulin resistance but also to the inhibition of melatonin and growth hormone, which aid in sleep and immune function, as well as repair.

Another big benefit of fasting for 12 to 16 hours is that it promotes autophagy, in which cells (including those in the brain) recycle components and destroy damaged proteins and mitochondria—which is good for renewal. Fasting also depletes the liver's stores of glycogen, a storage form of glucose, which is helpful because this helps push you into ketosis. Finally, fasting induces ketosis. It is best to break the fast with water (no ice) with some lemon, as a detoxifying drink. (Lemon helps detoxify by several different mechanisms, such as stimulating your liver and providing vitamin C.)

4. *Ketoflex 12/3 helps you to prevent gut leak and optimize your microbiome.* For most people, this means avoiding gluten, dairy, and other foods to which you are sensitive, and which may contribute to leaky gut and thus cause inflammation. Once your gut is healed, optimizing the microbiome means using probiotics and prebiotics.

Now that you know the principles behind Ketoflex 12/3, here are the specifics:

1. *Make foods with a glycaemic index lower than 35 the bulk of your diet.* They won't raise your glucose and therefore do not require a significant insulin release. You can find a list of glycaemic indices for various foods at http://www.health.harvard.edu/diseases-and-conditions/glycemic-index-and-glycaemic-load-for-100-foods.[2] The majority of your diet should be comprised of vegetables: organic ("Dirty Dozen & Clean 15" is a site to guide selection priority—http://www.fullyraw.com/dirty-dozen-clean-15), seasonal, local, and non-GMO (non-genetically modified).

2. *Avoid fruit juices in favour of whole fruits (which include the fibre).* Fruit smoothies are fine, but don't make them too sweet (that contributes to insulin resistance). To cut the sugar, you can add vegetables such as kale or spinach. Since tropical fruits such as mango and papaya have the highest glycaemic indices, opt for those with lower glycaemic indices, such as berries. The best fruits are wild, colourful berries, lemons, limes, tomatoes, and avocados (yes, tomatoes and avocados are, strictly speaking, fruits). As whole fruits (not

juices) are still high in nutrient density and fibre, they *can* be used as a dessert at the end of a meal containing dietary fat. Ancestrally, fruits were consumed at the end of summer to fatten for the winter. Avoid tropical fruits because of their increased glycaemic index.

3. *Avoid the "Berfooda Triangle."* Corny, I know, but by analogy to the Bermuda Triangle, which is dangerous for boats and planes, the Berfooda Triangle is a particularly damaging triad of food: simple carbohydrates, saturated fats, and lack of fibre (both soluble and insoluble). Think cheeseburger, fries, and soft drink. The lack of fibre leads to higher absorption of carbohydrates, which trigger inflammation and raise insulin levels. Therefore, if you plan to eat carbs, have kale (or another source of fibre) first! Eating fibre is a powerful way to reduce blood sugar—the carbohydrate absorption is curtailed and the optimal microbiome is supported. As for saturated fats, as noted above, they are wonderful for helping to induce ketosis, but when these are combined with simple carbohydrates and an avoidance of fibre, it's the perfect storm, producing cardiovascular disease, insulin resistance, and dementia.

4. *Avoid gluten and dairy as much as possible.* Although only 5 per cent of the U.S. population has marked gluten sensitivity, such as that causing coeliac disease, gluten can damage the gut lining in most of us, leading to leaky gut and chronic inflammation, among other problems. As for dairy, many of us can "handle" the inflammation it causes (and, after all, what is better than pizza?). But leaky gut and inflammation are two of the thirty-six holes in the roof we want to patch—two of the factors tipping the synapse preserving/destroying balance toward the latter. We don't want to leave a single hole unpatched. Cyrex Array 3 can show if you have gluten sensitivity. When you look for

gluten-free alternatives, just be careful not to choose any with rice flour or other high-glycaemic-index ingredients. You don't want to trade leaky gut for diabetes.

5. *Reduce toxins by eating specific detoxifying plants.* By toxins, I mean the hundreds we are exposed to daily, from heavy metals to endocrine-disrupting agents like BpA (bisphenol A) to biotoxins like trichothecenes. As it happens, the molecules in certain edible plants use multiple mechanisms to sequester and eliminate toxins from our bodies via urine, sweat, and stool. These detoxifying plants include coriander, cruciferous vegetables (cauliflower, broccoli, various types of cabbage, kale, radishes, Brussels sprouts, turnips, watercress, kohlrabi, swede, rocket, horseradish, broccli raab, rapini, daikon, wasabi, pak choc), avocados, artichokes, beets, dandelions, garlic, ginger, grapefruit, lemons, olive oil, and seaweed.

6. *Include good fats in your diet, such as those from avocados, nuts, seeds, olive oil, and MCT oil.* One approach, used successfully by some members of the website ApoE4.info, is to use MCT oil until you restore your insulin sensitivity. Then, since MCT oil is saturated fat and therefore on the "eat less" list for those with ApoE4, switch over to polyunsaturated fatty acids such as those in olive oil and other cold-pressed oils, or monounsaturated fatty acids such as those in nuts.

7. *Avoid processed foods in favour of whole foods.* Simple rule: If ingredients are listed, it's processed. As food writer Michael Pollan points out, if your grandmother would not recognize something as a food, you probably should not be eating it. Processing introduces many damaging molecules, from high-fructose corn syrup to carcinogenic dyes to neurotoxins such as acrylamide. Fresh, local, sustainable, organic vegetables avoid these toxins.

8. *Fish are optional.* Ketoflex 12/3 is, after all, flexitarian. Just keep in mind there are both advantages and disadvantages to fish. On the positive side, fish are an excellent source of omega-3 fats and other beneficial compounds, as well as protein. On the negative side, some fish contain high levels of mercury and other toxic compounds. Avoid large-mouthed, long-lived species such as sharks, swordfish, and tuna, since these are the highest in mercury, in favour of SMASH fish (salmon, mackerel, anchovies, sardines, and herring). Whenever possible, get wild-caught, not farmed, fish, which offer a better omega-3 to omega-6 ratio and fewer toxins.

9. *Meat is a condiment, not the main course.* Men need about 50 to 70 grams of protein each day and women about 40 to 60 (as noted above, one gram of protein per kilogram of weight is plenty, and in fact, some like to reduce to 0.8 grams per kilogram). Much beyond that may contribute to our carbohydrate burden by a process called transamination. Remember, you can get protein from food other than meat, such as beans, soy, eggs, and nuts. If you eat meat, try to get free-range chicken or grass-fed beef, because these preserve a good omega-3 (anti-inflammatory) to omega-6 (pro-inflammatory) ratio, thus reducing their inflammatory character. Eat small amounts (60 to 90 grams—"condiment" size—a few nights per week). Similarly, eggs should be from free-range chickens, not battery-raised, because such eggs also preserve a healthy omega-3 to omega-6 ratio.

10. *Probiotics and prebiotics should be included.* After healing your gut (described below), you need to optimize the bacteria there, which includes feeding the right bacteria (probiotics) with the right bacteria food (prebiotics). You can get both probiotics and prebiotics in pill form, but even better are

dietary sources. For the probiotics, those include fermented foods such as kimchi, sauerkraut, sour pickles, miso soup, and kombucha. Yoghurt also contains probiotics, but since it also has sugar (both through its lactose and, often, through added sugar) and of course is a dairy product, it is best to avoid it.

It is often helpful to include in your diet a yeast called *Saccharomyces boulardi*, which functions as a probiotic, especially if you have diarrheoa. Rather than destroying microbes (for example, with antibiotics), we want to optimize the microbiome—in the gut, on the skin, in the sinuses, and elsewhere. *Saccharomyces boulardi,* which is available in capsule form or powder, is particularly helpful if you have another yeast, such as *Candida,* which is part of gut dysbiosis, leading to symptoms such as bloating and gastric distress. Similarly, whenever you undergo treatment with antibiotics, it is important to follow that with probiotics and prebiotics to repopulate your microbiome.

For the prebiotics, the idea is simple: choose the food for the bacteria that you want to support (such as the *Lactobacillus* and *Bifidobacterium*), and avoid foods for the bacteria you want to keep out of your gut (such as some of the Firmicutes, which have been linked to chronic illnesses such as diabetes, inflammatory bowel disease, and metabolic syndrome). Prebiotic foods include jicama (Mexican yam), onions, garlic, raw leeks, raw Jerusalem artichoke, and dandelion greens.

11. ***Digestive enzymes are helpful.*** If you follow the Keto-flex 12/3 programme and eat a mostly plant-based diet, you are unlikely to experience acid reflux. But if you do, if your lab values indicate inflammation, if you are under chronic stress, if you have reduced stomach acid or are older than 50,

it is often very helpful to take digestive enzymes—available in capsules—with meals. It is also helpful to include digestive enzymes when switching from a carbohydrate-rich diet to a good-fat-rich one, since these enzymes help you to metabolize fat.

12. *Optimize nutrition and cognitive protection with supplements.* I recommend the following daily for everyone with cognitive decline or risk for cognitive decline, unless their laboratory values are optimal for each parameter:

- Vitamin B_1, 50 mg (as noted above, vitamin B_1 is important for memory formation)
- Pantothenic acid, 100–200 mg (especially if focus or alertness is an issue)
- The B_6/B_{12}/folate combination as described above for those whose homocysteine is above 6.
- Vitamin C, 1 g, for those with suboptimal vitamin C levels or who have copper:zinc ratios greater than 1:2.
- Vitamin D, starting with 2500 IU per day (or use the 100 x rule described earlier), until serum levels reach 50 to 80.
- Vitamin E as mixed tocopherols and tocotrienols 400–800 IU, for those with vitamin E levels less than 13.
- Vitamin K_2 as MK7 100 mcg, for those taking vitamin D.
- Resveratrol 100 mg, for all.
- Nicotinamide riboside, 100 mg, for all.
- Citicoline, 250 mg twice per day, to support synaptic growth and maintenance.
- ALCAR (acetyl-L-carnitine), 500 mg, to increase levels of nerve growth factor, especially for those with any contribution from type 2 Alzheimer's.
- Ubiquinol, 100 mg, to support mitochondrial function in everyone.

- Polyquinoline quinone (PQQ), 10 to 20 mg, to increase mitochondrial number for everyone.
- Omega-3 fatty acids (more on these below in the section on inflammation).
- Whole coffee fruit extract (WCFE), 100 mg once or twice per day for three months, then withdraw slowly over one month. This increases BDNF (brain-derived neurotrophic factor), and is especially important for those with type 2 (atrophic) Alzheimer's disease.

13. *Specific herbs support synaptic function.* I recommend the following, available as encapsulated extracts or as the herbs themselves, every day unless otherwise indicated:

- Ashwagandha, 500 mg, twice per day with meals. This helps in the reduction of amyloid, as well as in handling stress.
- *Bacopa monnieri*, 250 mg, twice per day with meals, to improve cholinergic function, one of the brain's key neurotransmitter systems (ashwagandha and bacopa are also available as nasal drops called Nasya Karma; if you prefer this to capsules, take 3 drops per nostril daily).
- Gotu kola, 500 mg twice per day with meals, to increase focus and alertness.
- *Hericium erinaceus* (lion's mane), 500 mg once or twice a day, to increase nerve growth factor, especially for those with type 2 Alzheimer's disease.
- Rhodiola, 200 mg once or twice per day, for those with anxiety and stress.
- Shankhpushpi (also spelled shankhapushpi and also known as skullcap), taken as 2 or 3 teaspoons or 2 capsules per day, to enhance branching of neurons in the hippocampus.

- For those with type 3 (toxic) Alzheimer's disease, MCI, or SCI, *Tinospora cordifolia* (guduchi) is helpful to boost immune support. It is taken at a dosage of 300 mg with meals, 2 or 3 times per day. Along with boosting immune support, those with type 3 may consider guggul, which removes toxins in the gut (somewhat like charcoal). This is typically taken as capsules of guggul extract, 350 or 750 mg per day.
- For those with type 1 (inflammatory) Alzheimer's disease, MCI, or SCI, or with bowel symptoms, triphala—a combination of amalaki, haritaki, and bibhitaki—is useful to reduce inflammation. This is best taken on an empty stomach, either as a capsule or by making a tea from the powder.

14. *Avoid damaging your food when you cook it.* The goal is for the food to taste good, while minimizing the loss of nutrients and the production of AGEs (advanced glycation end products). AGEs are glycotoxins created by a reaction between sugars and proteins or lipids. High levels create oxidative stress, inflammation, and many of the pathologies we see with diabetes and other chronic diseases.

Moist heat, shorter cooking times, lower temperatures, using acidic ingredients such as lemon, lime, and vinegar, and food choices (uncooked plants have no AGEs; uncooked animals do have AGEs) are all methods that reduce AGEs. Grilling, searing, roasting, and frying will produce AGEs.

What do you do if you are following the Ketoflex 12/3 diet and exercising, yet your fasting insulin remains over 4.5 or your hemoglobin A1c remains over 5.5 per cent or your fasting glucose remains over 90? No problem: several over-the-counter supplements target each. These should be introduced only one at a time, then followed up to determine the effects on glucose control and insulin sensitivity. For instance:

- Insulin sensitivity is affected by zinc levels, so if yours is below 100, try 20 mg to 50 mg of zinc picolinate daily, then recheck your glucose after two months.
- High hemoglobin A1c reflects poor glucose control, which is affected by low magnesium. If your RBC magnesium is less than 5.2, try magnesium glycinate (500 mg per day) or magnesium threonate (2 g per day).
- Cinnamon turns out to be a wonderful way to improve glycaemic control. You need only ¼ teaspoon each day, sprinkled on food, or you can easily take it as 1-gram capsules. Cinnamon also improves lipid profiles in people with type 2 diabetes.[3]
- Alpha-lipoic acid is an antioxidant. Most people use 60 mg to 100 mg daily.
- Chromium picolinate also lowers blood glucose, and 400 micrograms to 1 milligram daily is the typical dosage.
- Berberine lowers blood glucose, and is usually taken at 300 to 500 milligrams three times per day.
- Your doctor may also prescribe metformin to reduce blood glucose.

The Many Advantages of Regular Exercise

Have you heard? Sitting is the new smoking! We lead our lives sitting at computers, sitting in class, sitting in movies, sitting in our cars, sitting in meetings, sitting on the sofa watching television or playing games on our phones. We are sitting ourselves to death! Research has shown not only that exercise is beneficial, but that sitting is detrimental to cognitive and physical (especially cardiovascular) health. The most relevant benefits of exercise for cognition:

1. Exercise reduces insulin resistance, which as you now know is a key player in Alzheimer's disease.
2. It increases ketosis, which, among other effects, increases production of the neuron-supporting molecule BDNF.
3. It increases the size of the hippocampus, a key region for memory and one that shrinks in Alzheimer's disease.
4. It improves vascular function, which is crucial for neuronal and synaptic health.
5. It reduces stress, a key trigger of Alzheimer's-promoting inflammation.
6. It improves sleep, another necessity for cognitive health.
7. It increases the survival of newborn neurons that are created in the brain process called neurogenesis.
8. It improves mood.

What is the optimal exercise for cognition? You want to combine aerobic exercise, such as jogging or walking or spinning or dancing, with weight training, preferably at least four or five days per week, for 45 to 60 minutes in total each day. Work up to this slowly, stretch out, and take care of your joints! Of course, with the reduction of inflammation that comes with this protocol, your joints should actually do very well.

Some people like to work with a trainer, and others with a health coach, while still others prefer to exercise on their own. All are fine. If you are having trouble getting started, ask a trainer, family member, or friend to help you get started.

The Promise of Sleep, Delivered

It is a badge of courage to work late into the night. Years ago, as an intern in medicine and a resident in medicine and then neurology, I was sleep-deprived for five full years, regularly staying up more than forty hours at a stretch. My reactions were slowed, my judgement was impaired, my learning and memory suffered, my adrenaline increased, my stress levels never abated, and I would fall asleep at the drop of a hat, a few times even while evaluating patients. When I finished my residency, after a few weeks of "regular" existence, I felt as if a fog had begun to lift: my thinking was becoming clearer once again. So it is with cognitive decline: to avoid or reverse it, optimal sleep is indispensable.

A few years ago, I was talking to a behavioural neurologist who is an expert in Alzheimer's disease evaluation and clinical research. She explained that it is a mystery why some patients with MCI seem to improve, whereas many go on to develop Alzheimer's disease. When I asked whether she saw any differences between those who continued to decline and those who improved, she thought about it for a few moments. "Yes," she said, "the ones who get good sleep are the ones who tend to improve."

Hmmm, maybe it's not such a mystery?

Here's how to optimize your sleep, thus improving brain function:

1. *If your evaluation identified sleep apnea, it is critical to treat this.* For some people, a simple dental appliance is effective. Others may require a CPAP (continuous positive airway pressure) machine. Either way, having appropriate oxygenation and airway pressure during sleep are very important, not just for cognition but also for cardiovascular health, preventing gastroesophageal reflux (GERD), and

reducing the likelihood of obesity and pulmonary disease, among other benefits.

2. *Try to get as close to eight hours of sleep per night as possible, without using sleeping pills (which can compromise cognitive function).* Your brain normally produces melatonin at night, but only if it is dark—any exposure to light turns off your melatonin. As we age, our production of melatonin declines. Many people find that they sleep better and awaken more refreshed if they take physiological amounts (meaning amounts comparable to what the brain produces) of melatonin at bedtime—anywhere from 0.3 mg to 0.5 mg. If you need more than this, it's fine to take up to 20 mg. With the appropriate dose, you should awaken refreshed and may notice some increased dreaming. If you take too much, you may sleep well for a few hours but then awaken in the middle of the night, unable to fall asleep again. In that case, simply reduce the dosage. It is a good idea to take an occasional melatonin "holiday" (for example, skip one night per week). This allows your body to continue to make its own.

Melatonin is not a sleeping pill, so you won't feel the sedative effect that you would with benzodiazepines such as Xanax, which have been associated with risk of cognitive decline. With melatonin you are creating renewing, physiological sleep, whereas with sleeping pills you are simply turning down the voltage and drugging the brain.

One of the most common complaints of people with sleep problems, and a contributor to cognitive decline or risk for decline, is middle-of-the-night awakening. This has many potential causes, including menopause and hormonal imbalance (especially low progesterone), depression, stress, or gastroesophageal reflux. If you find yourself ruminating—fixating on one idea or unable to stop going over problems in your mind—you may get relief by taking tryptophan (Trp) at bedtime (500 mg). You can instead take 5-hydroxytryptophan (100 or 200 mg), since 5-HTP enters the brain more readily than Trp. If you are already on an SSRI (selective serotonin reuptake inhibitor) antidepressant such as Prozac or Zoloft or their generic forms, then you should avoid both Trp and 5-HTP. The combination of the antidepressant and the Trp or 5HTP may lead to serotonin syndrome, which is marked by fever, agitation, sweating, and diarrheoa. It occurs when the antidepressant prevents the uptake of the neurotransmitter serotonin from brain synapses, leaving it there and stimulating brain cells. Production of serotonin increases because of the greater availability of its precursor, tryptophan. This "perfect storm" is like plugging all the storm drains prior to a major cloudburst: it's a dangerous combination that causes flooding—in the case of your brain, flooding of the synapses with serotonin.

Another common cause of awakening in the middle of the night is reduced progesterone, which can affect both women and men. During perimenopause, it is common for levels of progesterone to drop relative to levels of oestradiol, with the result that the ratio of oestradiol to progesterone is too high. Since progesterone has a relaxing effect, loss of progesterone is associated with anxiety, poor sleep, and often "brain fog." If your lab tests show that your progesterone levels are suboptimal, ask your doctor about bioidentical oral progesterone, starting with 100 mg before bed. "Bioidentical" means that the hormone has the exact same molecular structure as the ones your body makes. In men, low progesterone levels are often associated with low testosterone, since progesterone is a precursor for testosterone. Since low testosterone is also a risk factor for cognitive decline, men should optimize their testosterone levels in coordination with their doctor.

Gastroesophageal reflux (GERD) is unlikely if you follow Ke-toflex 12/3, but if you do have GERD, it is important to avoid PPIs, proton pump inhibitors such as lansoprazole (Zonton Fastabs). You need your stomach acid to allow your enzymes to break down your food so that it can be absorbed properly—along with zinc, magnesium, vitamin B_{12}, and other essentials. Further-more, if you are making stomach acid appropriately, this should actually *inhibit* GERD, since the acid causes the lower esophageal sphincter to close, preventing reflux.

If you are awakening due to stress, consider meditation or a recording such as Neural Agility ("meditation on steroids"). Listening to this programme drives brain frequencies that are associated with relaxation and enhanced synaptic plasticity, the physiological basis for the formation of new memories. In order to use this approach you simply relax each evening (typically five nights per week), lie down, dim the lights, use a set of headphones, and play the programme using an iPhone or iPod or computer or other device for thirty minutes. You may feel some modest caffeine-like stimulation the first few days, but this should give way rapidly to a more relaxing effect.

If you had told me a decade ago that as a biomedical scientist, I would be recommending meditation, I would have laughed. But I cannot argue with research showing that people who are regular practitioners of meditation actually have increases in hippocampal volume, as well as other benefits such as reduced stress levels.

3. *Practise good sleep hygiene.*

- Keep the room as dark as possible (light reduces the mel-atonin that your brain normally makes during sleep), using a sleep mask if needed.
- Keep your environment as quiet as possible. Turn off

electronics and stay away from EMFs (electromagnetic fields), which are produced by televisions, video recorders, and other electronics.

- Wind down prior to sleep—going from high-pressure work straight to bed is asking for problems in falling asleep!
- Go to bed before midnight, if possible. Attempts at sleeping late to make up for late bedtimes are often thwarted by noises (phones, traffic, etc.), light, and other disruptions.
- Avoid exercise for a few hours before bedtime, since exercise ramps up your adrenaline and prevents sleep.
- Exercise early in the day, so that the adrenaline surge has calmed down before you go to bed.
- Avoid blue light, the kind in our standard lights (especially in the new LED lights), at night. Use filters for your reading light or computer if you wish to read on a device before bed.
- Avoid stimulants such as caffeine after early afternoon.
- Keep the television out of the bedroom.
- Avoid heavy evening meals.
- Keep hydrated, but don't drink so much water close to bedtime that you awaken in the middle of the night for a bathroom run.

The Surprising Effects of Stress

Stress refers to running a system at a level beyond where it was meant to operate. We humans did not evolve to lead the lives most of us lead—lives of sugar-laden diets, late nights with incandescent lights, constant anxiety about work, poor sleep, poor nutrition, and exposure to hundreds of toxic chemicals, to name just a few of the stressors pummelling our brains and bodies. We evolved to handle intermittent stress, not constant stress.

Stress increases levels of cortisol, which at high levels is toxic to our brains—in particular to the memory-consolidating hippocampus, which is one of the first structures to be assaulted by Alzheimer's disease. Stress also increases a number of risk factors for cognitive decline and Alzheimer's disease, including blood glucose levels, body fat, risk for obesity, carbohydrate craving, leaky gut and the resulting inflammation, permeability of the blood-brain barrier, calcium release and hyperstimulation of neurons, and the risk of cardiovascular disease. It also attacks factors that protect against Alzheimer's—the synapse-preserving ones that struggle not to be overcome by the synapse-ravaging factors, such as neurogenesis and the growth and maintenance of the dendritic spines associated with memory formation.

Stress is a factor in most cases of cognitive decline, but an especially strong one in type 3 (toxic) Alzheimer's disease, MCI, or SCI. For these individuals, stress worsens cognition especially rapidly. The onset of cognitive decline in such patients often coincides with a period of great stress.

> A HARD-DRIVING 56-YEAR-OLD LAWYER TOOK ON THE most difficult case of his career and worked on it nonstop for two years, with little sleep. He had been depressed for several years before. He won the case, but soon began to struggle to find the right word while speaking or writing and also had difficulty with calculations. He became passive and slow. His PET scan was strongly suggestive of Alzheimer's disease. He was ApoE2/3, not ApoE4. His lab values all pointed to type 3 Alzheimer's disease: TGF-β1 and C4a were both increased, for instance, and he had signs of mycotoxins in his nose and throat.

That's why it is critical to include stress reduction in the programme for cognitive optimization. The best approach will vary from person to person. For many people, meditation and yoga are powerful stress reducers, lowering cortisol, protecting the hippocampus from atrophy, and increasing the thickness of the cerebral cortex.

The simplest—but surprisingly rarely used—approach to stress reduction is to take a few deep, slow, diaphragmatic breaths (breathing from your belly, not your chest). Relax!

If you feel hyper after exercising, dial it back—maybe 30 minutes instead of 45, or a slower treadmill pace. You still want to get your heart rate up and do some weight training, but if you are stressing out with marathon training, then cutting back may help lower cortisol.

If you are a caffeine junkie, cutting back may help your stress levels. That also goes for alcohol. Massages, laughter, music, movement—these are all wonderful ways to reduce stress.

Brain Training

The idea that mental exercises—usually computer-based—can improve cognitive function has been controversial, with some scientists criticizing unproven hyped claims. But let's not throw the baby out with the bathwater. Hundreds of scientific papers have shown important cognitive effects of brain training. For example, one speed processing training programme called Double Decision reduced the risk for dementia by nearly 50 per cent ten years after the training, which is far more than any drug ever has.

Many companies provide online brain training, including Posit Science, Lumosity, Dakim, and Cogstate. The leading expert in this field is Professor Mike Merzenich, founder of Posit Science, which makes BrainHQ. In 2016 Mike won the prestigious Kavli Prize for Neuroscience for his groundbreaking work in the area of neuroplasticity. I have been listening to Mike's brilliant lectures since the 1980s, and there is no argument that his group is years ahead of everyone else in this field, with over 130 papers demonstrating the benefits of BrainHQ.

The BrainHQ group has optimized the programmes so you need only 10 or 20 minutes per day, five days per week, to see improvements. Alternatively, you can use a schedule of 30 minutes, three times per week. Start with Hawkeye and Double Decision, and you can add memory and other processing speed games, but don't get discouraged! The programmes are set up to continue to challenge you, so as soon as you start doing well, they become more difficult. Relax, and if it's too stressful, simply cut back on the time.

Inflammation

Inflammation is one of the most important drivers of cognitive decline, and it feeds directly into the Alzheimer's disease mechanisms. Resolving inflammation is therefore critical to reversing cognitive decline. Once your lab tests have determined *why* inflammation is present, I recommend a three-pronged approach to reducing it.

1. *Resolve the inflammation.* An effective way to do this is by taking supplements called specialized pro-resolving mediators (SPMs). SPMs, with names like resolvins, protectins, and maresins, are produced by the body at the site of inflammation and act as resolution agonists, helping the immune response complete its response to infection or other inflammation-triggering threat and return to the baseline healthy, noninflammatory state. If the body is not doing this on its own, SPM supplements can provide the missing resolution agonists. You can take two to six capsules per day, for one month. During this time, it is important to remove the underlying cause(s) of the inflammation, such as poor dietary habits and chronic infections.

2. *Inhibit new inflammation.* Anti-inflammatories such as omega-3 and curcumin help prevent new inflammation. I recommend one gram daily of the omega-3 DHA

(docosahexaenoic acid), from fish oil or krill or algae, and the same amount of curcumin, either on an empty stomach or with fats. There are many other anti-inflammatories, such as ginger, cinnamon, pregnenolone, cloves, thyme, as well as anti-inflammatory foods such as green leafy vegetables, beets, and broccoli. The ReCODE protocol does not include non-steroidal anti-inflammatories such as ibuprofen because they can damage the gut and kidneys.

3. *Remove all inflammatory sources.* It isn't much good to treat inflammation if you also keep triggering it, so it is critical to prevent exposure to inflammagens. There may be more than one source, including leaky gut, a diet high in either simple carbohydrates or trans fats, and chronic infections such as from Lyme disease, viruses such as *Herpes simplex*, or moulds such as *Aspergillus* or *Penicillium*. Poor oral hygiene can also cause chronic inflammation; as noted earlier, oral bacteria such as *P. gingivalis* have been found in the brains of Alzheimer's patients.

If inflammatory markers remain high after removing these obvious potential contributors, then you should get a more complete evaluation. It should check for autoantibodies, such as those that cause rheumatoid arthritis, chronic Lyme disease, other tick-borne infections such as *Babesia* or *Bartonella,* and other undiagnosed medical conditions.

Healing the Gut

There are several ways to heal the gut. There are whole books and websites on this, but I'll summarize the key points.

Healing the gut is critical for most of us, since leaky gut is so common. If your Cyrex Array 2 is positive or you have food sensitivities, bloating, constipation, or loose stools, you likely have leaky gut, meaning that the integrity of your gut lining has been compromised. Healing your gut reduces systemic inflammation, improves nutrient absorption, enhances immune responses, and supports an optimal microbiome, thus increasing the products of the microbiome, such as some hormones and neurotransmitters. It is a key tactic in the prevention and reversal of cognitive decline.

The first step to healing the gut lining is understanding the causal insults, then eliminating or minimizing these. Here is a list of the potential triggers:

- Sugar
- Allergy/sensitivity to gluten (or other grain allergens), dairy, or other foods
- Allergy/sensitivity to chemicals such as those found in processed foods (sodas, artificial sweeteners, preservatives, dyes, binders, and so on)
- Herbicides (such as glyphosate)
- Pesticides
- GMO foods (genetically modified organisms)
- Alcohol
- Antibiotics—orally or in animal-based foods sourced from CAFOs (concentrated animal feeding operations)
- Anti-inflammatories—such as aspirin or other NSAIDs (non-steroidal anti-inflammatory drugs like ibuprofen), or steroids
- Stress

In addition to eliminating or minimizing these potential insults to the gut, there are complementary measures for gut healing. One method is bone broth,[4] which is safe and physiological. In fact, many ancestral and traditional cultures that consume minimal meat—such as the Okinawan people, who are known for their longevity—are very assiduous in their use of animal bones, providing a source of cartilage, tendons, and bone marrow that release collagen, many amino acids such as glutamine and glycine, minerals, and vitamins that seal the gut and thus strengthen the intestinal barrier.

Many of these cultures would keep a pot simmering all day and use the broth as a base for their soups, stews, and other dishes. Some groups advocate drinking bone broth for a period of time ranging from one day to three weeks while eliminating, then reintroducing, foods one at a time. Others use bone broth as an adjunct to the Ketoflex 12/3 diet (see Julie's protocol in Chapter 9).

You can buy bone broth sourced from organic, pastured animals or wild-caught fish, or make your own. There are several excellent websites that discuss methods to purchase or make your own bone broth, such as http://scdlifestyle.com, https://www.kettleandfire.com, and https://chriskresser.com/?s=bone+broth.

If you don't find bone broth to your liking, there are workarounds, just as there are for most elements of ReCODE. Some people take colostrum capsules or L-glutamine capsules or zinc carnosine, all of which help heal the gut. Another approach is to follow a diet that uses specific carbohydrates to allow gut healing, called the SCD diet: https://draxe.com/ scd-diet.[5]

Regardless of whether you heal your gut with bone broth, colostrum, L-glutamine, or the SCD diet, after three to four weeks, your gut should be healing. Have yourself retested for leaky gut by the Cyrex Array or other method to make sure it is now healed. If it has indeed healed, you can now include probiotics and prebiotics in your diet. (If you take probiotics when your gut is still leaky, you run the risk of leaking the bacterial fragments into your bloodstream, increasing the inflammation.) This is something like cleaning and repairing your leaky fishbowl (healing your gut), which allows you to add fish (the probiotics) and fish food (the prebiotics).

As noted in the section on nutrition above, the best way to do this is with foods. Basically, you get your probiotics (bacteria) from fermented foods such as sauerkraut and kimchi, and your prebiotics from fibre-rich foods such as jicama (Mexican yam), onions, leeks, and garlic. If you do take a probiotic capsule in addition to these foods, you want to use a probiotic that contains 30 billion total cfu (colony-forming units, which represent live bacterial counts) to 50 billion cfu. Dr. David Perlmutter, a neurologist and the author of *Brain Maker*, recommends including the five core species of bacteria listed in Table 3.

Once you have optimized your gut microbiome, you should experience no bloating, constipation, or diarrheoa, and you will have removed an important source of inflammation. You will also eliminate toxins more efficiently, and most important, you will have taken a major step toward improving cognition.

Table 3. Five core species of bacteria recommended for probiotics[6]

Species	Effects	Source(s)
Lactobacillus plantarum	Regulates immunity, reduces gut inflammation; maintains nutrients.	Kimchi, sauerkraut, other fermented vegetables
Lactobacillus acidophilus	Immune enhancement, reduces yeast infections, improves cholesterol.	Fermented dairy
Lactobacillus brevis	Increases BDNF, improves immune function.	Sauerkraut, pickles
Bifidobacterium lactis	Reduces food-borne pathogens (e.g., Salmonella), enhances immunity, improves digestion.	Fermented dairy
Bifidobacterium longum	Reduces pathogens, improves cholesterol.	Fermented vegetables and dairy

Now that your gut is healed and your gut microbiome optimized, it is time to address another and—where cognitive decline is concerned—potentially even more important microbiome: the rhinosinal microbiome in your nose and sinuses. As any cocaine user will tell you, the quickest way to the brain is through the nose. Microbes have also figured this out,[7] and we are finding many examples in which the nose, throat, and sinuses are affected by chronic rhinosinusitis (inflammation of the nose and sinuses). The culprits are often mould species and/or bacteria such as MARCoNS (Staph bacteria that form protective coatings called biofilms and are resistant to many antibiotics). Biofilms are "bacterial igloos" that shield bacteria from antibiotics, making them much more difficult to eradicate.

It is not only the sinus and nasal microbiome itself that has access to the brain. So do the products the microbes secrete, which can destroy molecules in the brain that support neurons and synapses. Therefore, if your lab results indicate an increase in C4a (this is a component of your immune system that goes up with exposure to biotoxins), if you have symptoms suggestive of type 3 Alzheimer's disease, or if you have chronic sinus problems, it is important to address the microbiome of your sinuses and nasopharynx. The approach is simple and stepwise. For additional information, you may wish to consult Dr. R. Shoemaker's website, http://www.survivingmold.com, or to be evaluated by one of the doctors certified in Dr. Shoemaker's protocol, as listed on his website.

1. *First, if pathogens such as MARCoNS (multiple antibiotic-resistant coagulase-negative Staph) or mould are present, they should be treated.* For MARCoNS, a nasal spray called BEG—Bactroban (mupirocin) 0.2 per cent, edetate disodium (EDTA) 1 per cent, and gentamicin 3 per cent)—is effective. It can be combined with SinuClenz and Xlear to

reduce burning and help healing. You can treat mould species with itraconazole, an antifungal, or the immune enhancer guduchi (*Tinospora cordifolia*).

2. ***Restore an optimal microbiome.*** There are products coming out to do exactly that—probiotics for the nose and sinuses, including ProbioMax ENT and Restore. (Restore was originally developed for gut health, but now also has a nasal formulation.) If you can't find them, a workaround to restore your nasal microbiome is to swab your nose with kimchi juice. The point is the same as with your gut microbiome: protective microbes prevent the reappearance of damaging ones like MARCoNS.

3. ***Remove the source(s) of pathogens.*** If there are moulds in your home, car, workplace, or any place else you spend a lot of time, you need to remove these. A company such as Building Forensics (https://www.buildingforensics.co.uk) can assess an area for mould and give you an assessment of the problem and suggest solutions practical if the mould is at your workplace, so in that case you would of course want to talk with the administration. Not surprisingly, this is a controversial area, but there are an increasing number of well-documented mould-associated illnesses, including cognitive decline, from both workplace and home exposures.

Hormonal Balance

Reaching optimal hormone levels is one of the most effective and most critical parts of ReCODE, but it is also one of the most controversial and difficult to optimize, for several reasons. First of all, the use of hormone replacement (HRT) by postmenopausal women is still hotly debated. Some experts argue against HRT for almost all women, while others say it should only be considered in the first five years after menopause, and still others contend that it should be considered in women who have Alzheimer's, MCI, or SCI, even if they are in their seventies, eighties, or nineties. Therefore, it is important to consult an expert in bioidentical hormone replacement, preferably one who has experience with cognitive decline. Again, the reason I emphasize bioidenticals is that these hormones have the same molecular structures as the ones made in your body, meaning they are more likely to produce the same benefits, and less likely to produce unwanted side effects. Bioidentical oestrogens are 17 beta-oestradiol, oestrone, and oestriol. Non-bioidentical oestrogens are, for example, those in the urine of pregnant mares, which is the source of the drug Premarin.

As with levels of vitamins and other compounds, and as discussed earlier in the section on the treatment concepts, "within normal limits" may bear little relationship to what values are optimal. This is of course especially important when you are optimizing cognitive function and reversing cognitive decline. Therefore, the goal is not to get you "within normal limits," but rather to get you to the optimal value for each hormone.

A third issue is that measured hormone levels do not tell us how the hormone is functioning in your body, only how much there is. In order for you to benefit from any hormone, the hormone needs to reach its receptor, bind to the receptor, travel with the receptor into the nucleus, and turn on many different genes that produce proteins that will exert their coordinated effects on your metabolism. You can see how many, many steps there are between the measured hormone levels and the actual effects of each hormone! This is why it is important to bookend the evaluation—that is to say, to look at the hormone levels as an upstream measure and the symptoms as a downstream measure. For example, when evaluating thyroid status, you can get a good analysis of the actual thyroid function by evaluating basal body temperature in the morning, or using *Thyroflex* to measure the timing of one of your reflexes. If your temperature is not at least 97.8 degrees Fahrenheit (36.5 degrees Celsius), then your thyroid function is likely to be suboptimal. Moreover, if there are clear thyroid-related symptoms such as weight gain, lethargy, constipation, or hair loss, thyroid function is likely suboptimal.

A fourth challenge is that the function of the hormones must be considered not simply individually but also in concert, since they affect each other. So one must look not at thyroid function in isolation, but at its interactions with other hormone systems such as the adrenal glands and the sex steroids. Optimizing all of these allows the whole system to work at its best, and this includes supporting your best cognition.

In order to prevent or reverse cognitive decline, it is critical to work with your doctor to optimize hormone levels:

1. *Thyroid:* As noted above, thyroid function is suboptimal in many people with cognitive decline. The major active thyroid hormone is T3, but the usual treatment is T4 (levothyroxine), which may or may not be converted efficiently to T3. Therefore, it is preferable to take the combination of T3 and T4 found in thyroid extracts such as Armour Thyroid or NP Thyroid or Nature-Throid or similar preparations. If you prefer to use synthetics, then you may need to combine levothyroxine with liothyronine. Tracking your symptoms and labs will help to optimize the dosage. In addition, since producing your own thyroid hormone requires iodine, if your thyroid levels or function are suboptimal, check your iodine level. If it is low, take iodine pills (one daily) or a source of iodine such as kelp.

2. *Oestradiol and progesterone (for women):* Oestradiol (and, to a lesser extent, related oestrogens, oestrone and oestriol) and progesterone have powerful effects throughout the body, including the brain. It is for this reason that

treatment with oestradiol and progesterone is controversial. On the one hand, oestradiol and progesterone have brain-protective effects, beneficial cognitive effects, and a direct effect on the molecular balance that drives Alzheimer's disease. It was for this reason that oestrogen was evaluated as a potential therapeutic for Alzheimer's disease (not surprisingly, it was not by itself found to be helpful). On the other hand, oestradiol can also, especially without the balancing progesterone, increase risk for uterine cancer and breast cancer. Therefore, if your levels of these hormones are low, confer with an expert in this area who is experienced in treating cognitive decline and risk for cognitive decline.

There are several key points to discuss with your expert practitioner:

- There is increasing agreement that bioidentical hormones— ones that are identical to those made by your own body— are preferable to imitators such as Premarin.
- There is no consensus on how long after menopause it is appropriate to treat a woman who is experiencing cognitive decline or who is at risk for it.
- Different practitioners employ different target values for oestrogens, and the optimal value for the reversal of cognitive decline as part of an overall programme is unknown. Some argue that the goal is 80 to 200 pg/ml (80 is the threshold for preventing osteoporosis), whereas others suggest that 30 pg/ml may be enough. There is also disagreement about whether to measure oestradiol in saliva, in 24-hour urine samples, or through other methods.
- For progesterone, start with 100 mg or 200 mg of a bioidentical such as Utrogestan, at bedtime. The target is 1 to

20 ng/ml, but monitor your symptoms (such as mood swings and lethargy), which may indicate that your progesterone levels are too high, to optimize your oestradiol to progesterone ratio.

Take the bioidentical oestradiol (or oestradiol-oestriol combination) transdermally or transvaginally, since taking it orally can lead to liver damage. And be sure to monitor your cognitive response, as well as your hormone levels and any side effects. Since HRT has been shown to increase the risk of breast cancer, keep up with mammograms (at a frequency appropriate for your age) and gynoecological exams such as cervic smear tests.

For reasons that are not yet completely clear, it is especially important for women with type 3 SCI, MCI, or Alzheimer's disease to optimize their hormone levels. In fact, many type 3 patients trace the onset of their cognitive changes to menopause or perimenopause. Therefore, if you have characteristics of type 3 Alzheimer's, please discuss bioidentical HRT with your physician.

3. *Testosterone is another critical player in the synaptic minuet, and optimal levels support synaptic maintenance.* If you have cognitive decline or are at high risk for it, it's a good idea to consult your physician about optimizing testosterone levels.

For men: This is especially so if your total testosterone level is below 300 ng/dL or your free testosterone level is below 6 pg/ml (for men; for women, the target levels are much lower, of course, and women should have total testosterone levels in the 30 to 70 range). Like other hormones, this is a powerful molecule, with effects in the brain and throughout the body. Therefore: (1) Work with your physician to keep your levels optimal, taking testosterone gel or cream if they are too low, or one of the testosterone-increasing supplements readily available. (2) Monitor for side effects, such as following your PSA (prostate-specific antigen) for prostate cancer and your calcium score or treadmill for cardiovascular disease. (3) Monitor your cognitive response and use the minimum effective dose. (4) Do not go off testosterone cold turkey if you want to discontinue; wean yourself off supplements slowly, over a few months, since the sudden mismatch between levels of the hormone and numbers of testosterone receptors is damaging, causing synaptic loss and associated cognitive decline.

Women too can benefit from optimizing testosterone, with the lower level targets, as noted above.

4. *Adrenal function—cortisol, pregnenolone, and DHEA:* When you are stressed, your adrenals kick into gear, producing something of a double-edged sword. On the positive side, the stress response is protective against pathogens and other threats; on the negative, high cortisol levels damage hippocampal neurons. You want the Goldilocks solution: levels of adrenal hormones that are not too high, not too low, but just right. Since pregnenolone is the master steroid, from which oestrogens, testosterone, and cortisol (among others) are derived, if you are under stress, you may "steal" the pregnenolone to generate cortisol, reducing your ability to produce oestradiol or testosterone. This "pregnenolone steal" is fairly common. It can be addressed through over-the-counter pregnenolone supplements starting at 10 mg daily and then moving up to 25 mg or whatever boosts you to a pregnenolone level of 50 to 100 ng/dL.

If your morning cortisol is low (less than 8 mcg/dL), you should undergo further evaluation, since this may be a sign that you respond poorly to stress. Similarly, if your morning cortisol is high (over 18 mcg/dL), you should undergo further evaluation to determine whether there are important unrecognized stressors such as ongoing infection.

> FOR TWO YEARS LISA, 52, HAD COMPLAINED OF DIFFICULTY with memory and word finding. She accidentally left the hob on, causing a fire. She had a strong family history of Alzheimer's disease. Neuropsychological assessment suggested a diagnosis of amnestic MCI, and her MoCA score was 25/30, also compatible with MCI. She had multiple suboptimal hormone levels. Her physician sent her to an endocrinologist, who unfortunately dropped the ball:
>
> 1. He did not check Lisa's basal body temperature or even ask about it; nor did he use Thyroflex, so he had no idea about her actual thyroid function.
>
> 2. Lisa's free T3 was very low at 1.8, but her free T4 was fine at 1.3. Her TSH was very high at 5. This combination means she was not converting T4 (the precursor of T3) to T3 effectively, a common problem, and the increased TSH showed that her body was recognizing a low-thyroid state. The endocrinologist simply increased her T4 and added no T3, which shows he did not understand her problem: since she was not converting T4 to T3, and T3 is required as the active thyroid hormone, simply increasing T4 is not the solution.
>
> 3. Her pregnenolone was very low, but he said that this is "just a pro-hormone" and therefore unimportant to address. In fact, pregnenolone has important effects on brain function.
>
> 4. He did not optimize her oestradiol or progesterone, indicating that he did not understand the absolutely critical effects of estradiol and progesterone on cognition.

Metal Homeostasis

Medical dogma holds that Alzheimer's disease is not caused by metals such as mercury, infections, hypothyroidism, low levels of vitamin D, or apparently, anything else. As I explained in chapter

4, however, there is clear evidence that cognitive decline, including Alzheimer's disease, is caused by an imbalance between synapse-preserving and synapse-destroying processes, and that dozens of factors can decrease the former and accelerate the latter, in many cases by acting directly or indirectly on APP (amyloid precursor protein). The evidence is clear that APP responds to metals such as iron, copper, and zinc.

BETH, 70, COMPLAINED OF MEMORY LOSS. SHE DEMON-strated deficits in short-term memory, word-finding, and comprehension, and had difficulty with technological devices such as her iPhone, and got confused trying to find her way even in familiar places. Her ApoE genotype was ApoE3/4, her FDG-PET scan had the marked hypometabolism in the temporal and parietal lobes that characterizes Alzheimer's, her amyloid PET was positive (also compatible with Alzheimer's), and her MRI showed hippocampal volume at only 18th percentile for her age. Her inorganic and organic mercury levels were high, with the total mercury at the 95th percentile. Her excretion of mercury was markedly below normal, a likely contributor to her mercury toxicity.

In medical school, we are taught to distinguish Alzheimer's disease from "reversible causes of dementia." This idea is fundamentally flawed, however, because the reversible causes of dementia are themselves potential contributors to the very process we refer to as Alzheimer's disease. Beth (above), Karl (from chapter 6), and many others have symptoms and scans that reflect true Alzheimer's disease, and mercury is a contributor. That's not the case in most patients with Alzheimer's disease, but it is in an important minority. That makes it crucial not to miss signs of mercury toxicity, especially since it is readily treatable.

If your mercury (especially inorganic mercury) is high, it is helpful to have your amalgams removed by a biological dentist—one trained to remove the amalgams without exposing you to high levels of mercury in the process. It is best to do this slowly, one or two at each appointment until they have all been removed. It is also important to remove the mercury from your system. One effective method, developed by Quicksilver, is gentler than heavy chelation: it uses pulsed treatments that activate a gene called Nrf2, helping your body eliminate mercury, lead, arsenic, iron, and other potentially toxic metals.

If your ratio of copper to zinc is high (both should be about 100 mcg/dL, and thus the ratio should be about 1), you should take steps to raise your zinc levels and lower your copper levels until the ratio falls below 1.3:1. Professor George Brewer, whose research I mentioned in chapter 7, has shown that treating zinc deficiency and copper overload lead to cognitive improvement. He recommends the following:

1. Zinc picolinate, 25 mg to 50 mg (but no more than 50 mg) each day to boost zinc
2. The antioxidant alpha-lipoic acid, 30 mg to 60 mg each day (to prevent oxidative damage associated with increased copper)
3. Vitamin C, 1 g to 3 g daily (to chelate and remove copper)
4. Pyridoxine (vitamin B$_6$) 100 mg daily (to enhance detoxification)
5. Manganese 15 mg to 30 mg each day (to support antioxidant enzymatic effects)
6. Stress reduction
7. The avoidance of vitamins with high copper contents

Also, check your inflammatory markers (such as hs-CRP), since chronic inflammation contributes to both high copper to zinc ratio and cognitive decline.

Toxins

Detoxification may be the most difficult part of ReCODE, since there are so many toxins that can contribute to cognitive decline. Fortunately, there are many therapeutics available when it comes to detoxification, starting with food.

CAROL, A 59-YEAR-OLD NURSE, HAD BEEN EVALUATED AT A nationally renowned Alzheimer's centre for cognitive decline every year for four years. Her initial neuropsychological evaluation suggested MCI, her MRI showed severe hippocampal atrophy to below the 1st percentile for her age, and her ApoE genotype was 3/4. She was treated with memantine but continued to decline, developing Alzheimer's disease. Not surprisingly, she became quiet and slow to respond, uninterested in reading or engaging in conversation.

When her husband brought her to see me, I explained that she had type 3 Alzheimer's disease (based on her age at onset, symptom complex, and laboratory values), and thus was highly likely to have had some toxic exposure. Tests showed very high levels of mycotoxins in her urine, as well as Lyme disease (and subsequent tests showed the common Lyme coinfection *Babesia*). She also had high levels of IgG, indicating hypersensitivity to *Cladosporium herbarum*, *Penicillium notatum*, and pigeon droppings. Her MARCoNS culture was positive. Her home ERMI score (this is a score for mould; average for all homes is zero) was 6.7, indicating high levels of toxic mould.

Carol began the ReCODE protocol. To address the mycotoxins, she received intravenous glutathione twice per week. With each administration, she showed clear improvement, but by the next morning she had regressed. She also received cholestyramine and intranasal VIP, as part of the Shoemaker Protocol for mycotoxin exposure. She moved into a new home, but unfortunately its ERMI score was 7; she began to spend more time outdoors and in a motor home. She also obtained a mobile HEPA filter to use when she was indoors. She began to improve. After six months her husband wrote, "Carol is now much better. She has been able to follow conversations and give very appropriate responses. Most noticeable has been a return of personality and social interaction. She worked on CMEs (continuing medical education) and was able to interpret and find answers better than she has in a long time. She was so excited about it that she continued for hours."

To get a clue about whether you have been exposed to high levels of toxic substances, start with your history:

- Have you had general anaesthesia? If so, how many times?
- Do you eat fish with high mercury content, like tuna, swordfish, or shark? How often?
- Do you have mould in your house, car, or workplace?
- Do you eat processed or nonorganic foods?
- Have you had tick bites?
- Do you take any medications?
- Do you take proton pump inhibitors (PPIs) for acid reflux?
- How much alcohol do you drink?
- Do you use makeup, hair spray, or antiperspirant?
- How often do you sweat? (It's an important route for toxin elimination.)
- Are you constipated? (Bowel movements are another route for toxin elimination.)
- Do you drink at least 32 ounces of purified water daily? (Urination is a third important route.)

A MAN CONTACTED ME ABOUT HIS 52-YEAR-OLD WIFE, who had been suffering cognitive decline for two years, starting at menopause. She had been prescribed sertraline (Lustrol) for possible depression. She had difficulty writing cheques, paying bills, and completing sentences. Her PET scan was strongly suggestive of Alzheimer's disease. When asked about mould exposure, her husband said, "No . . . well, except for all of the black mould in the basement, but I assume that is not a problem."

If you have metal toxicity—especially high levels of mercury or a high ratio of copper to zinc—there are several ways to treat it, such as chelation. A gentler but equally effective method, as noted in the discussion about metal homeostasis, is that from Quicksilver, called the Detox Qube.

If you have toxicity due to toxins from mould or other microbes—biotoxins—as indicated by the tests and values described above, the optimal treatments are somewhat complicated and exposure-specific. It is therefore helpful to work with a physician—ideally, one experienced in the treatment of biotoxin-associated illness, such as those certified in the Shoemaker protocol[8] or functional medicine physicians experienced with biotoxin illness.[9]

1. First, if the tests in chapter 7 show that you harbour pathogens such as MARCoNS or mould species, your doctor should treat them as described in the discussion above on the sinus microbiome.

There are several ways to inactivate and excrete pathogen-associated biotoxins, and increase cognition in type 3 Alzheimer's, MCI, or SCI:

- Intravenous glutathione, which is a powerful antioxidant and antitoxin, may bring a rapid improvement in mental status, but it typically lasts only a few hours. Nevertheless, twice-weekly infusions can lead to sustained gains in cognition. Alternatively, you can increase glutathione with liposomal glutathione, nebulized glutathione, or N-acetylcysteine capsules.
- Intranasal VIP (vasoactive intestinal peptide) provides trophic support to the brain. It is typically administered once

MARCoNS cultures are negative. These administrations are often associated with cognitive improvement.

- Certain foods enhance detoxification. They include coriander, cruciferous vegetables (cauliflower, broccoli, various types of cabbage, kale, radishes, Brussels sprouts, turnips, watercress, kohlrabi, swedes, rocket, horseradish, broccoli raab, daikon, wasabi, and pak choi), avocados, artichokes, beets, dandelions, garlic, ginger, grapefruit, lemons, olive oil, and seaweed.

- You can increase how quickly you eliminate toxins by binding the toxins in your gut with cholestyramine, Welchol, or guggul (or, especially for metals, *Chlorella*); and by enhancing excretion via sauna followed by showering with a non-emollient soap (e.g., Castile); and by urination following hydration with filtered water.

- Patients with biotoxin-associated illness often improve most when their protocols include bioidentical hormone optimization.

2. Second, after treatment, restore an optimal microbiome by following the steps listed above for probiotics for the nose and sinuses.

3. Third, remove the source(s) of pathogens. If visual inspection or an ERMI score indicates there are moulds in your home, car, or workplace, you have several options. One is to spend more time outdoors, though obviously there is a limit to that unless you want to become a full-time camper. Alternatively, you can purchase a mobile HEPA filter, which are widely available. I recommend Dr. Ritchie Shoemaker's excellent book on biotoxins, *Surviving Mold,* for tips on how to do this.[10]

CHAPTER 9

Success and the Social Network: Two People's Daily Routines

Success is how high you bounce when you hit bottom.
—GEORGE S. PATTON

JULIE, ONE OF the many people who has done extremely well on ReCODE, was kind enough to share her daily routine. She has been on the programme for five years, so it has evolved as various risk factors have been addressed and is now quite extensive, but don't let that discourage you. As I said earlier, each person's protocol is unique, optimized for his or her situation, and you can adopt elements of the programme one at a time.

JULIE HAD BEEN SHOCKED TO FIND THAT SHE WAS HOMOZY-gous for ApoE4, and had already developed significant cognitive problems at only 49, becoming lost in familiar places, failing to recognize faces, and losing her memory. Until her genetic test, be-cause of her age she had not even considered the possibility that she was developing Alzheimer's disease. Unfortunately, one of her cousins then developed severe Alzheimer's disease, starting at an even earlier age. Julie called a neurologist who specializes in Alzheimer's, and after waiting months for an appointment was finally able to see him. She explained her genetic and symptomatic status, asking him to help her to avoid further decline, and, if possible, restore her memory and cognition to what it had been. Brusquely he said, "Good luck with that," offering no hope whatsoever (sadly, we neurologists are not, as a group, known for our bedside manner). Julie soon found that she was not alone. There are about 7 million Americans who carry two copies of the ApoE4 allele, and more than 99 per cent do not know it. Another 75 million Americans have a single copy of ApoE4. As you might imagine, learning your ApoE status when you have already begun the process of cognitive decline is heartbreaking.

Julie's cognitive evaluation showed her to be at only the 35th percentile for her age when she started treatment. However, after several months on the programme, she noted marked improvement, and her cognitive evaluation rose to the 98th percentile. It remains there five years (and counting) later. Julie has been extremely attuned to changes in her ability to think and remember, and has taken note of what seemed to help and what seemed to bother her. I have heard this repeatedly from people who have done very well.

Here is Julie's daily routine, with thanks to Julie for sharing it with everyone:

- I wake up, ideally without an alarm (not always possible!) after 7 to 8 hours of sleep.
- I skip breakfast and enjoy a cup of organic coffee, no cream, with a very small amount of 100 per cent pure stevia. This is a necessity for me. I experience both enormous cognitive and mood benefits from a small amount of coffee.
- If I feel very hungry (rare for me) I'll take a 1000 mg MCT (medium-chain triglycerides) capsule in the AM to help me get into ketosis. [She uses a ketone meter (details in Appendix B) and tries to keep her blood level of ketones in the range from 0.5 mmol/L to 2 mmol/L. The ketone meter measures beta-hydroxybutyrate, one of the three so-called ketone bodies. This

mild ketosis is induced by fasting, exercising, and eating a diet very low in carbohydrates and high in good fats.]

- I use the Ayurvedic practice of oil pulling with coconut oil for 5 minutes, then brush my teeth with a nonfluoride toothpaste [oil pulling has been done for centuries; it reduces decay-causing bacteria, whitens teeth, and improves the oral microbiome].
- I try to avoid any toxins in my cosmetics or toiletries. I use an aluminum-free sunscreen and deodorant. I've stopped using nail polish and use coconut oil instead. In an effort to use the safest products, I check all of my toiletries and cosmetics against the Environmental Working Group's Skin Deep database: http://www.ewg.org/skindeep/.
- I take fish oil (that includes 1000 mg DHA) and curcumin prior to exercise, which I do to increase BDNF [brain-derived neurotrophic factor, which supports neurons and has an anti-Alzheimer's effect].
- I walk/run for 50 to 60 minutes every single day—even in very inclement weather with the proper gear. I find very hot, cold, wet, snowy, windy weather to be invigorating. By challenging myself, I become stronger. Spending time in nature is also very healing and grounding for me.
- While I walk, I often listen to meditative music.
- Sometimes, I challenge myself with cognitive tasks while I walk. I try to say the alphabet backward, count backward from 100 by nines, eights, sevens, etc.
- Prior to officially breaking my fast, I drink a glass of room temperature water with lemon and/or ginger to detoxify.
- I eat my first meal of the day after noon, ending a 15- to 16-hour fast.
- A typical first meal for me would be two pastured (high omega-3) eggs with a huge plateful of colourful local, organic nonstarchy vegetables. Broccoli, spinach, kale, and fermented vegetables are always among my core choices. I also include a few sweet potato wedges or raw carrots for the vitamin A. I liberally use high-polyphenol EVOO (extra-virgin olive oil) to finish my vegetables, along with dried sea vegetables for the iodine and pink Himalayan salt, fresh herbs and spices to season.

- I floss and brush my teeth again (I repeat this after each meal).
- I take the remainder of my "morning" supplements, which include vitamin D_3 and K_2 (I'm very careful to take these two with dietary sources of vitamin A and fat to increase solubility and bioavailability). I also take ALCAR (acetyl-L-carnitine), citicoline, ubiquinol, PQQ (polyquinoline quinone), ginger, and a small divided dose of NAC (N-acetylcysteine) and alpha-lipoic acid (I repeat these last two in the PM). Additionally, I take vitamin B_1 (thiamine) to assist with glucose homeostasis and methylcobalamin, methylfolate, and P5P (pyridoxal-5-phosphate) to keep homocysteine low. I also take a VSL#3 probiotic.
- As I work at my desk, I remind myself to stand up and walk around for 10 to 15 minutes of every hour. When I'm working from home, this is a great opportunity to do household chores—laundry, sweeping, dishes, pulling weeds, raking, etc. I have learned to reframe "chores" as being positive as they enable me to be very active. Being grateful for the work also helps me keep a positive attitude.
- I take a twice-weekly yoga class, which is very helpful for strengthening, balance, and centring. I try to practise daily.
- I sip organic Japanese green tea and one cup of bone broth (fat removed) throughout the day, but refrain from snacking.
- I strategically time my resveratrol and NAD supplementation to upregulate SirT1 in order to get the best benefit. Some evidence suggests that they may interfere with the benefits of exercise when taken around the same time. Through personal experience, I've learned that they interfere with sleep if taken before bed. I've settled on early to mid-afternoon (several hours after exercise) when I can still benefit from the energy boost.
- I usually take a mid-afternoon break from work and challenge myself to a 20-minute brain training session. I use both Lumosity and Brain HQ. Switching them up keeps it fresh for me. I try to keep this fun and nonstressful. My goal is to try to match or beat my score from the previous day.
- I like to meditate after brain training. Just emptying my mind for 15 minutes has proven invaluable.

- I eat my second meal between five and six p.m. Dinner typically consists of wild-caught fish (Alaskan sockeye salmon is a favourite). I enjoy this with an enormous salad consisting of many mixed greens, red cabbage, avocado, nuts, seeds, and a wide variety of nonstarchy vegetables. I use pink Himalayan salt, sea kelp granules, and fresh herbs and spices to season along with a high-quality balsamic vinegar, lemon, and lots of high-polyphenol EVOO (extra-virgin olive oil). I sometimes enjoy a very small amount (60 ml) of a dry red wine, like cabernet.
- After dinner, I like to walk again with my husband or a friend, socializing with neighbours along the way. I also enjoy kayaking on our lake after dinner.
- Several times per week, I indulge in dessert. I enjoy raw organic walnuts and sliced almonds, with coconut flakes and a few wild organic berries drizzled with unsweetened kefir (from A2 cows) with a small amount of 100 per cent stevia to sweeten. Another treat would be a dark chocolate square (86 per cent or higher cacao).
- I stop eating by seven p.m. and try to get to bed by ten. Several hours before bed, I put on my blue blocker glasses. I try to dim lights at this time and refrain from exercise or stimulating work or conversation. I also use a programme on my laptop, phone, and tablet that blocks blue light.
- I take my evening supplements an hour or so before bed. These include magnesium citrate (magnesium threonate is too sedative for me), ashwagandha, and melatonin. I also take a small dose of NAC (N-acetylcysteine) and alpha-lipoic acid along with a different probiotic—MegaSporeBiotic.
- I use my topical testosterone and oestrogen in the evenings (along with a twice-weekly transdermal oestrogen patch) and an oral dose of progesterone every PM.
- Because my husband is an airline pilot and often works odd hours, I sometimes sleep in a separate bedroom when he has to wake up very early or comes home in the middle of the night.
- I darken the bedroom completely before sleep. Any source of light can interfere with melatonin production. All electronic devices in my bedroom have radiation shields and are placed on

airplane mode before sleep. I also keep the bedroom cool and put essential lavender or rosemary oil on the bedsheets to aid in relaxation and promote healthful sleep.

Please do not worry—there won't be a quiz on this! Furthermore, it is important to realize that each protocol is personalized, so this may not be the optimal one for you. And remember, you need not start every element of your protocol at once. Also, it will not interfere with any drugs that you may have been given for cognitive decline. In fact, if anything, it should make them more effective. The key, however, is to get started as early in the process as possible, preferably as soon as symptoms appear, or as soon as you learn that you are at risk for cognitive decline, whether through genetic testing, family history, blood tests, or imaging.

Here, for comparison, is the ongoing programme for Kelly, who has also shown marked improvement after experiencing difficulty getting lost, difficulty with memory, and with working. As you'll see, however, Kelly is doing several of the components suboptimally and has not included several recommended components (and has been somewhat obstinate about considering the suggested improvements to her protocol!). The key point is not that she is doing things optimally—she is not there yet—but that she has followed her own cognition, and if/when this declines, she will once again optimize. Of course, I believe that she could do still better if she would optimize her programme now, but I have not yet convinced her about this, and she is doing very well!

Here is Kelly's regimen:

- Seven to eight hours of sleep each night, taking 3 mg melatonin before bed, and 500 mg tryptophan (which reduces ruminations if you awaken in the middle of the night). She uses her phone sleep monitor to measure how much sleep she is getting.

- Twelve-hour fast each night.
- Aerobic exercise for 30 to 45 minutes each day, six days per week.
- Yoga for 60 to 90 minutes, five times per week.
- Transcendental meditation for 20 to 30 minutes, two times each day.
- A gluten-free, low-glycaemic, mostly plant-based diet. She drinks coffee and, occasionally, red wine.
- Kelly takes hormone-replacement therapy (HRT), but this is not bioidentical: 2.5 mg medroxyprogesterone orally every other day and 2 mg oestradiol orally (oestradiol should be taken transvaginally, not orally, because of potential liver toxicity, as well as improved levels with transvaginal delivery).
- 88 mcg levothyroxine (T4) each day, and one extra on Saturdays. (This is fine as long as the conversion from T4 to the active T3 is efficient. For many people, however, simply taking the relatively inactive T4 is not optimal.)
- 3000 IU fish oil daily.
- 2000 IU vitamin D3 daily. (Any dose over 1000 IU should be accompanied by 100 mcg to 250 mcg vitamin K_2.)
- A daily multivitamin.
- 500 mg citicoline daily.
- 2100 mg curcumin daily. (This should be taken on an empty stomach, or with good fats, for absorption.)
- 250 mg *Bacopa monnieri* daily (best taken twice per day).
- 1000 mg ashwagandha daily.
- Probiotics and 3 tablespoons nutritional yeast.

Kelly is not doing any brain training or strength training, is taking suboptimal hormone-replacement therapy (oral rather than transvaginal, bioidentical oestradiol), may be taking a suboptimal thyroid treatment, is not taking iodine (in some people, the low thyroid is simply because of iodine deficiency), and has not been evaluated for innate immune system activation so does not know whether this is contributing to her cognitive changes. She is not taking resveratrol or magnesium threonate, is not checking to determine whether she is in mild ketosis, and is not taking MCT oil. However, what she is doing has for her worked very well, and as long as she monitors her own status and optimizes the programme if/when her improvement dissipates, she should be fine.

As you can tell from the fact that Kelly is doing well without following every single facet of ReCODE, some is better than none, but all is better than some.

I mentioned that Julie is homozygous for ApoE4—that is, she carries two copies of this genetic variant, the most important genetic risk factor for Alzheimer's disease, and so has ten times the risk of developing Alzheimer's as the general population does. She founded the social networking website, ApoE4.info, which includes people from all over the world who discovered, through genetic testing, that they carry the ApoE4 gene (either heterozygous or homozygous—that is to say, one copy or two). They had all heard the dogma that there is nothing that can delay, prevent, or reverse Alzheimer's disease, and many felt hopeless and alone. They began to chat online several years ago, then founded ApoE4.info.

On the website, people share and discuss research, communicate with experts, compare advice and strategies, and even conduct what they call "n = 1 experiments"—meaning they try something on themselves (the 1) and share with others how something like tracking biomarkers and following particular protocols worked for them. Most of all, they share any shards of information that might possibly, even against their own doctors' claims, be helpful. Members, who post anonymously under a handle, help each other to read and interpret the large medical literature on Alzheimer's disease and ApoE4.

When Archimedes, in the third century BCE, said, "Give me a long enough lever and a place to stand, and I will move the Earth" (not in English, of course!) he probably did not realize that the twenty-first-century version of his proposed lever would be constructed of silicon and electrons and the collective synaptic network of billions of nervous systems. Nonetheless, I think he would agree that social networking is truly moving the Earth. And I have seen that it can move people to take control of their cognitive fate in ways they might not have used had they not been part of a social network.

In May 2015, ApoE4.info members met in person for the first time, at the Buck Institute for Research on Aging. Many were already on the protocol I had published several months before. After a few lectures, we sat around a large table in a glass-enclosed room just off the atrium, each member in turn telling his or her story: the hanging of crepe by doctors, the complete confidence with which experts declared there is no effective treatment for Alzheimer's, the desperation of family members, the helplessness of the patients and potential patients (most of the ApoE4 carriers were not yet showing signs of cognitive loss). It was one of the most remarkable events I have ever witnessed, poignant and yet hopeful, as people identified themselves by their screen name: "I am Go Girl," or "I am Lost at C." Others would erupt, "Oh, *you* are Go Girl!" or, "Oh, *you* are Lost at C!" having read many of the other's posts. Tears flowed, heads shook. But for the first time, hope sprang, as people shared their stories of improvement.

ApoE4 members got together again in August 2016 at the Ancestral Health Symposium in Boulder, Colorado. I attended, too, and it was emotional and inspiring. Almost all of the nearly 600 members of ApoE4.info were on some variation of ReCODE. Again, they shared personal histories; again, they described their initial hopelessness upon learning their ApoE4 status. One of the members, an academic scientist, told the group she had joined the website a few months before, heard the many success stories, and so was quite sanguine about her problems. She didn't feel hopeless or terrified about her future. She said she knew of a number of people who had done very well on the programme, and therefore had every expectation that she would be fine.

We were on the fifth floor of the Memorial Building of the University of Colorado. It was a beautiful August Saturday. I took a deep breath and closed my eyes for a moment. Here was a woman who was not afraid of Alzheimer's disease, not because she was uninformed or tranquillized or detached or resigned, but because she was analytical and intelligent. She was aware of the successes of numerous people in ApoE4.info, the similarity of her genetics to theirs, and therefore was appropriately, and understandably, optimistic.

The number one concern of individuals as we age is the loss of our cognitive abilities; for those so stricken, progression to severe dementia has been to date an ineluctable future, with nothing but bad news from every expert source. The social network, with its continued evaluations and comparisons and analyses, along with the personalized programmatics approach, the larger data sets, and a collective determined optimism—all of these had colluded to begin to change medical history. It was a moment written into my synapses, one that I will never forget.

Social networking is the key to a world without dementia. Comparing notes, gathering information, identifying problems and iterative enhancements, detecting unsuspected issues, sharing successes, encouraging prevention, empowering patients and presymptomatic individuals—these are all catalyzed by social networking. What the several hundred members of ApoE4.info have done can and should be scaled to the hundreds of millions worldwide who would benefit from similar connectivity and activism.

POSTSCRIPT: I HEARD from Julie today, who told me that the ApoE4.info website now includes approximately 800 members, that "about 99 per cent" are on some variation of the protocol, and that they are hearing repeated stories of improvement. That call made my day.

PART FOUR

Maximizing Success

CHAPTER 10

Putting It All Together: You *Can* Do It

The secret of getting ahead is getting started.
—MARK TWAIN

THIS CHAPTER SUMMARIZES the ReCODE protocol, boiling it down to the essentials to make it as easy as possible to use, and offering a table to which you can refer. As you'll see, it's pretty simple. All of the scientific details, all of the lab tests, and all of the treatment nuances detailed in the preceding chapters boil down to five key points that drive cognitive decline in nearly everyone. There is nothing that cannot be dealt with effectively:

1. Insulin resistance
2. Inflammation/infections
3. Hormone, nutrient, and trophic factor optimization
4. Toxins (chemical, biological, and physical)
5. Restoration and protection of lost (or dysfunctional) synapses

ReCODE: The Basic Plan

Intervention	Notes
Diet: Ketoflex 12/3	Target ketosis 0.5–4 mmol/L.
Exercise: aerobic and strength, 30–60 minutes, 5 to 6 times a week	Ramp up slowly, protect your heart.
Sleep: 7–8 hours; melatonin 0.5–3 mg; Trp if ruminations; sleep hygiene	Exclude sleep apnea.
Stress reduction: meditation or Neural Agility; yoga; music; diaphragmatic breathing	
Brain training: 30 minutes 3 times a week, or 10–20 minutes 5 to 6 times a week.	
MCT oil 1–3 g twice per day	When insulin sensitivity restored, can drop MCT and increase extra-virgin olive oil, monounsaturated fatty acids, and polyunsaturated fatty acids.
Curcumin 1 g twice per day (or turmeric)	On empty stomach or with good fats.
Ashwagandha 500 mg twice per day	With meals.
Bacopa monnieri 250–500 mg twice per day	With meals.
Gotu kola 500 mg once or twice per day	For alertness and focus.
Other herbs as indicated	See text re: rhodiola, hericium, shankhpushpi, triphala, guduchi, guggul indications.
Magnesium threonate 2 g per day	May be sedative, so take at night.
Ubiquinol 100 mg	
PQQ 10–20 mg	
Resveratrol 100 mg	
Nicotinamide riboside 100 mg	
Omega-3: DHA 1 g, EPA 0.5–1 g	
Liposomal glutathione 250 mg twice per day	
Probiotics and prebiotics	If leaky gut, heal gut first.
Vitamin D and vitamin K_2 (MK7)	Target D level of 50–80.
Mixed tocopherols and tocotrienols 800 IU	Target vitamin E level of 12–20.

Intervention	Notes
Bioidentical HRT	Optimize hormone levels, including thyroid, adrenal, sex hormones.
SPM (specialized pro-resolving mediators) x 1 month	If hs-CRP > 1.0.
Methylcobalamin 1 mg, methylfolate 0.8–5 mg, P5P 20–50 mg	If homocysteine >6; if B$_{12}$ <500.
Alpha-lipoic acid 100 mg, N-acetylcysteine 500 mg, cinnamon ¼ teaspoon, berberine 300–500 mg three times a day or metformin	If fasting insulin >4.5, or fasting glucose > 90, or hemoglobin A1c >5.5.
Zinc picolinate 25–50 mg, alpha-lipoic acid 100 mg, N-acetylcysteine 500 mg, P5P 50 mg, Mn 15 mg, vitamin C 1–4 g	If zinc < 80 or copper:zinc > 1:3.
SAM-e 200–1600 mg or folate 5 mg	If there is depression.
Consider huperzine A 200 mcg	After 3 months on the protocol, if memory is the primary problem and not on donepezil (Aricept).
CIRS evaluation and treatment (cholestyramine, intranasal VIP, etc.)	If evaluation indicates type 3 (high C4a, high TGF-β1, low MSH, etc.).
Detoxification protocol	If metals or biotoxins identified.
Specific antibiotics or antivirals	If infections identified.
Discontinue or minimize medications that interfere with cognitive function	For example, statins, PPIs, benzodiazepines, etc.

The summary is simple, but the implementation is the key—you can do this!

As more and more people have adopted ReCODE, I have been able to see which practices are associated with the greatest success. Some are obvious, while others are less so.

1. *The sooner you start, the better your chance for complete reversal and protection.* One woman told me she was not ready to start the protocol. "I'm fairly early in my symptoms," she said, "but when I'm further along, I'll contact you to get started." No, no, a thousand times no!! The earlier you start, the better, since the pathophysiological

process underlying Alzheimer's disease proceeds for decades. What may seem "early" with respect to symptoms is usually *not* early with respect to the ongoing disease process. Ideally, you would adopt the protocol as prevention. Pretty much everyone knows that, when you turn 50 years of age, you should have a colonoscopy. Well, when you turn 45, or as soon thereafter as you can, please consider the "cognoscopy" I described in chapter 7. Checking your genetics, biochemistry, cognitive function, and imaging (the imaging is optional if you have no symptoms) is relatively easy, and becoming more so. If you decide against prevention, then it's critical to obtain evaluation and treatment as early as possible, if and when cognitive decline begins. To date, every individual with subjective cognitive impairment (SCI) has improved on the protocol, so don't start any later than that.

2. *"Live your protocol" for at least six months.* Behaviour change is not easy, so don't beat yourself up if it takes you a while to implement the diet, sleep, and exercise regiments described above. It becomes easier after the first month or two. So hang in there! You really need to adhere to the protocol that addresses *your* situation for six months or so to see positive effects. Doing a bit here and there while ignoring much of it rarely helps.

LAURA WAS IN HER MID-SEVENTIES WHEN SHE BEGAN TO experience memory loss. Her mother had developed severe dementia, also in her seventies. Laura's evaluation revealed numerous metabolic abnormalities, including suboptimal hormone levels, increased homocysteine, and reduced vitamin B_{12}. All were readily addressable, and after several months on ReCODE she was markedly brighter and more responsive. However, she began to regress; it turned out she had discontinued various parts of the protocol.

When I discussed this with Laura and her family, she offered excuses and explanations. She said that she liked sweets and could not give them up, simply did not wish to exercise, and did not want to change her nutrition. A health coach spent hours with her, but she simply did not wish to adopt the protocol despite her early positive results. Her family was unable to change her mind, and she continued to decline.

Yes, changing your diet is difficult, especially since most people do not believe diet has such a profound effect on cognition and the risk of dementia despite the accumulating research—for example, on the Mediterranean diet—to the contrary. (When we began sending health coaches to visit people using the protocol, it turned out everyone was cheating on the diet!) Numerous behavioural changes are important for enhancing your cognition, and each has its own role to play, so be patient with yourself. We have found that health coaches are very helpful in getting people to make the requisite changes, as are supportive spouses, family members, and supportive practitioners.

3. *Identify what is wrong; don't treat blindly.* I am often asked what one thing is the most important in the protocol. Is it the nutrition? Hormones? Addressing inflammation? Or what? The answer is this: obtaining a thorough evaluation, as explained in chapter 7. Only then can you and your practitioner identify what is contributing to your cognitive decline. Furthermore, if your cognition does not improve on ReCODE within a few months, then you need to identify what is holding you back. Typically, from 10 to 25 lab values are suboptimal. Knowing which they are allows you to focus on the elements of ReCODE that specifically target them—and inspires you, too, I hope, not to skimp or cheat on those elements!

4. *Keep optimizing.* One of the main differences between

ReCODE and standard monotherapies (pills) is that you continue to optimize. Again and again, we find that tweaking the protocol based on lab values and responses brings continued cognitive improvement. This is especially true for people who are keenly aware of their cognitive status. Of course you can follow your status with online quantitative neuropsychological testing, including through BrainHQ, Lumosity, Dakim, or Cogstate, among others. Even after you have improved, test your lab values to see if any have fallen out of the optimal range, and test your cognition so you know how you're doing, every four to six months. This is a marathon, not a sprint, so keep optimizing. You may be surprised at the continued improvement in cognitive function.

5. *Be diligent about your lab values.* There is a threshold you need to cross so that synaptoblastic processes (preserving synapses, making and maintaining memories) outweigh synaptoclastic ones (destroying synapses and losing memories and cognitive function). When you are evaluated and the potential contributors to cognitive decline are identified, you won't know how many will have to be optimized to get you over the threshold so that synaptoclastic processes no longer outweigh synaptoblastic ones, There is as yet no direct way to measure where this threshold stands, and it might be different for different people. For now, it is therefore important to address as many of the suboptimal values as possible.

DIANE BEGAN TO HAVE MEMORY LOSS AROUND PERIMENO-pause, and it became quite severe following menopause. She responded very well to ReCODE. After a year, however, she noticed that her memory had started to get worse again, so she began to keep a diary of when her memory failed. Despite this setback, Diane did not return for re-evaluation immediately. When she did, it turned out that her oestradiol level had fallen from greater than 100 picograms per millilitre to 0. It turned out that her doctor had changed her oestradiol formulation from transvaginal (excellent absorption) to transdermal (often poor absorption). Her memory problems had appeared within a month of this change.

Sometimes the threshold is exceeded when specific hormones are optimized, sometimes when sleep is optimized, sometimes when intravenous glutathione is added, sometimes when stress is reduced, sometimes when mild ketosis is achieved. The point is to attend to detail. When you get it right, your metabolic parameters will show it, giving you the best opportunity for cognitive success.

6. *Do what you can—you don't necessarily have to follow every part of the protocol.* The good news is that, once you get over the synapse preserving/destroying threshold, you are in good shape. Patient Zero had superb results following twelve of thirty-six recommendations. That doesn't mean a limited palette will work for everyone. As long as there are contributors to cognitive decline, you are at risk, so try not to skip any elements of the protocol. However, addressing the most important contributors turns out to be good enough for many people.

7. *With each tweak of your protocol, try to notice over the ensuing days and weeks whether cognition gets better, worse, or neither.* Results that are temporally linked are not necessarily causally linked, but again and again it turns out that people whose metabolisms, lab values, and other measures respond to various parts of their own personalized protocols see excellent cognitive improvement, too, over the long haul. Also, remember that cognitive decline—indeed, neurodegeneration in general—is progressive: that is to say, it gets worse and worse. A lack of progression—in other

words, staying the same even if the same is less than ideal—is therefore often the first sign that you are on the right track. Even modest gains are a very good sign, because it means that you have stopped the decline, turned the corner, and are headed in the right direction.

8. ***Don't let the perfect be the enemy of the good.*** As long as you have high fasting insulin and insulin resistance, chronic inflammation, depleted hormones, or exposure to dementogens, your cognitive status is unlikely to get better. Your brain will continue to produce amyloid as a protective response to these threats, and amyloid unleashes the synaptic-destructive quartet. However, as all of these metabolic and toxic parameters begin to improve, and there is no further reason for your brain to produce amyloid, you should start to see cognitive improvement—even if your lab values still fall short of optimal. Let me show you how one patient, who had twenty-four metabolic and toxic abnormalities, did on ten months of ReCODE.

66M ApoE4/3	2014	2015 (ReCODE 10 months)
Fasting insulin	32	8
Hs-CRP	9.9	3
Homocysteine	15	8
Vitamin D$_3$	21	40
Symptoms	Struggling	Working full-time

Not only did this patient's cognition improve; his MRI also showed clear evidence of improvement. As you can see, that occurred along with his metabolic improvement, even though he had not reached the optimal levels: for example, his fasting insulin decreased from 32 to 8, whereas the optimal is 4.5 or lower.

Similarly, his hs-CRP, a key indicator of inflammation, fell from 9.9 to 3, but optimally should be below 1.0. His homocysteine dropped from 15 to 8, whereas below 7 is the goal. So follow your numbers to give yourself the best shot at cognitive health, but don't be discouraged if you don't hit the target right away: just heading in the right direction metabolically will point you in the right direction cognitively.

9. *Document your cognitive status so you know where you stand, when you are improving, and when things need to be adjusted.* Just as your lab values are indispensable in pointing you in the right direction for your therapeutic protocol, your functional status is invaluable in tracking your improvement or lack thereof. This can be done with standard quantitative neuropsychological testing, or online tests from BrainHQ, Lumosity, Dakim, Cogstate, or other brain-training companies. If you do not see improvement over time (months), then you need to make changes to your protocol, search for additional potential contributors to the cognitive changes, or both.

You can document your structural status using MRI with volumetrics, such as those offered by Neuroreader or NeuroQuant (currently, less than $100 and usually covered by insurance in the US). Volumetrics turn MRI into a very powerful tool for estimating atrophy in various brain regions.

10. *Take advantage of social networks.* It is often helpful to discuss your symptoms, issues, questions, and concerns with people in similar circumstances. This can be done in person or via the Internet, including in groups such as ApoE4.info.

11. *Be careful about going off therapeutics cold turkey.* In general, biological systems were not made to function like

spigots that you turn on and off quickly. If you are going to discontinue hormone replacement therapy or donepezil (Aricept) or thyroid hormone or any other therapies, taper off extremely slowly. With donepezil, for instance, sudden cessation may be followed by increased cognitive decline.

12. *Stick with the programme.* ReCODE offers many benefits, not just to cognition but also to metabolism, glucose control, weight, and detoxification. My hope, when the initial patients showed improvement, was that people would take years to show worsening if they ever discontinued the program. In other words, the underlying process had taken years to develop, so after patients showed improvement, I hoped that it would again take years for symptoms to appear once they had disappeared. That has not turned out to be the case, unfortunately. People who have gone off and on multiple times experience cognitive decline within two weeks. Going back on the protocol restarts the improvement, but from a lower baseline than if you stick to it.

We do not know why cognition declines so quickly when you drop the programme. Here is one possibility. When a country sends troops to a problem area, and the battle or war ends, it often leaves a policing force behind so any future problems can be stemmed rapidly. So it is with the immune system: even after you begin ReCODE it seems to leave behind amyloid troops produced to fight microbes or metals or toxins, even though ReCODE is eliminating the targets they had been fighting. The immune system seems to shelter amyloid in a biological fort (the amyloid plaques) so that they do not damage brain cells but are immediately available when needed. "Needed" can be when you stop following ReCODE and thereby allow the factors that damage synapses to build back up again. Result: plaques release amyloid molecules to once again fight the perceived threat—and amyloid, as we know, destroys synapses.

Whatever the underlying mechanism turns out to be, it is important to stick with the programme, and to continue to tweak and optimize over months and years.

13. *You don't need to start the whole programme at once; you can take it in phases.* It is easy to be overwhelmed by trying to start an extensive programme all at once, so don't worry! Your health coach, doctor, and family members can help you, adding one element and then another. If you want to start by optimizing your sleep and increasing your physical activity, putting off the dietary changes for a few weeks, that's fine. If you want to start the dietary changes by adopting the twelve-hour (overnight) fast first but postpone the hormonal optimization, that's also fine. Just be sure you eventually—ideally, within three to six months—adopt as many elements as you can. I promise that it will become easier over time.

Taking these keys to success into account, there are patterns in who responds the best. The best responders generally include the following:

- *People who are at risk, because of their ApoE status, but who do not yet have symptoms.* It will be years before we can be certain about how effective ReCODE is at prevention, but so far we have not seen anyone convert from asymptomatic to symptomatic while on the programme.
- *People with subjective cognitive impairment.* Similarly, to date, no one with SCI has failed to improve on the protocol.
- *People with early mild cognitive impairment.* In its early

stages, with MoCA (Montreal Cognitive Assessment) scores of 24 or higher, there is a better chance for improvement. Even people with scores as low as 1, which is associated with advanced Alzheimer's disease, have shown improvement, however. MCI tends to respond best if it is aMCI (amnestic MCI) and if there are identifiable suboptimal laboratory values.

- *People with early Alzheimer's disease.* Although we call this "early Alzheimer's disease," the underlying pathophysiological process has been present for two decades or so, indicating that this is late in the course of the underlying process. Nevertheless, we have had many people with early Alzheimer's disease, and MoCA scores in the teens or MMSE scores of 20 or high teens, show clear cognitive improvements.

Although earlier treatment produces better outcomes, we occasionally hear from people who have initiated the protocol late in the course of Alzheimer's disease and achieved at least some positive results. Here is an email I received in 2015.

Dear Dr. Bredesen,

I have recently moved from California to Oregon, where my wife and I are now living with, and caring for, my 82-year-old father-in-law. He is depressed and in a fairly advanced state of dementia, with good days and bad. He has been compliant in taking many ReCODE supplements and it has immediately lessened the worst of his depression and listlessness. Now he is more engaged in holding forth, telling stories of his glory days, over and over, a big improvement over sobbing and howling that he is confused and is not sure where he is. My point is that even if a person cannot be brought back to high functioning with the ReCODE protocol, the process of caring for a family member with dementia can be radically improved in a very short span of time using ReCODE. And it is far too early to judge how far he might improve.

- *Forms of cognitive decline—SCI, MCI, early Alzheimer's (AD)—that are not type 3 (toxic).* The type 3 subtype of AD has proven to be the most difficult to treat successfully, although even with this subtype, the earliest changes (SCI) are often readily reversible. However, once type 3 AD is recognized, the treatment becomes more complicated because the toxic source(s) must be identified and removed, any organisms involved must be dealt with, and the ongoing immune response must be quieted. We have nonetheless had success with some type 3 patients, in particular those with high levels of mercury. Treating that reverses cognitive decline fairly quickly, making this an exception to the usual results in type 3.

- *People with cognitive changes who are otherwise healthy.* Perhaps not surprisingly, those who are not on multiple medications for chronic illnesses tend to respond more completely to the protocol.

- *People who have no brain atrophy on MRI, or in whom the atrophy is restricted to the hippocampus.* When there is widespread brain atrophy, people typically have difficulty with understanding concepts, organizing, word finding, and more. They may also become more passive and childlike. This pattern occurs more commonly with type 3 Alzheimer's, although it may also occur late in other types. When this atrophy is absent, the response to the ReCODE protocol is in general more successful.

- *People who are younger than 75.* This is not to say that those 75 and over have not shown response, but in general, greater and more rapid responses have occurred in younger patients.

- *People who have supportive spouses and doctors.* Supportive spouses have proven to be remarkably helpful, and many have adopted the programme for themselves as well. They help in many ways, from aiding in compliance to reducing stress to helping patients find joy. Doctors who have trained in functional or integrative medicine and understand the networks and programmatic approaches to chronic illnesses also help enormously. On the other hand, doctors can be inflexible. Here is one of the thousands of emails I received following our first study showing reversal of cognitive decline.

Dear Dr. Bredesen,

We read your article on the reversal of cognitive decline and hoped to discuss the possibilities of this therapeutic programme with our family doctor. He dismissed it out of hand, saying he had no time to read. He would not even accept a copy of your article. When we asked for a referral to a doctor that might be interested in helping with this approach, he simply said, "Doctors don't do nutrition." The neurologist he had sent us to earlier said Aricept was the only solution, and that is not an acceptable solution to us. When we asked about homocysteine, eyes rolled.

What appealed to us about your programme is that the first six components are already in place. I have fibromyalgia that I can generally control through diet, exercise, and stress management (instead of medications).

On the other hand, ReCODE tends to be less effective for people who show no improvement in their laboratory values (which usually simply means that they have not followed the protocol), who do not attend to the details of the programme, who do not follow the programme diligently, who do not start until late in the Alzheimer's process, who do not include follow-up, who do not include continued optimization, who have severe type 3 Alzheimer's, and whose healthcare team works at cross purposes instead of pulling together.

I can't conclude this chapter without a confession. If someone had told me a few decades ago that, as a research neurologist, I would be recommending protocols that involve meditation, yoga, laughter, music, joy, fasting, exercise, herbs, nutrition, and sleep, I would have laughed. But I cannot argue with results, or with the conclusions of years of research. Indeed, my wife, an excellent family practice and integrative doctor, told me twenty-five years ago, during my laboratory's early research into neurodegeneration, that whatever we found would end up having something to do with basic processes such as nutrition, stress, and toxicity. Of course, since I took a reductionist approach, I argued that we would ultimately identify one specific molecule that would be the key to Alzheimer's disease. Needless to say, I should have listened to her.

CHAPTER 11

This Is Not Easy— Workarounds and Crutches

The floggings will continue until morale improves.
—OFTEN ATTRIBUTED TO CAPTAIN BLIGH OF THE BOUNTY

C APTAIN BLIGH'S PERHAPS apocryphal quote illuminates a paradox analogous to the very one involved with optimizing treatment for Alzheimer's disease, MCI, and SCI. Learning that, since stress is an important contributor to the pathophysiology of dementia, you must avoid stress—well, that puts a fair amount of stress on you, doesn't it? Add to that the suggestion that you must give up some of the foods that you love, and the stress at the prospect of adopting the ReCODE programme only increases.

STEVE, 73, HAD BEEN EVALUATED AT TWO MAJOR MEDICAL centres for cognitive decline that included difficulty with memory and attention, and had worsened over the past seven years. He had been told that he had probable Alzheimer's disease, and although no cerebrospinal fluid had been evaluated and no PET scan had been done, he turned out to be homozygous for ApoE3 (E3/3), to have clear evidence of leaky gut, gluten sensitivity, leaky blood-brain barrier, and multiple autoantibodies (including against his own brain tissue). When I explained this, he said, "Do you mean I have to give up pizza?!?"

Well, yes. Maybe not forever, but it certainly should not be a staple of your diet. Believe me, I know that this and other elements of ReCODE can be difficult for some people. But remember, if you find that despite what may seem like your best efforts, the programme isn't working for you, the most likely explanation is the obvious one: people try to skip parts of the protocol and leave out critical elements. Fortunately, in the years that I've worked with patients to help them adhere to the protocol, I've found crutches and workarounds for many of the elements they struggle with:

- "I don't want to give up ice cream."

Since it is best to avoid the inflammation-triggering dairy and sugar in ice cream, try coconut milk ice cream, which is dairy-free and has a low glycaemic index.

- "I'll be miserable if I give up chocolate."

No problem, just try organic dark chocolate with a high cacao content (over 70 per cent) and a low glycaemic index. Just don't overdo it: my patients tell me a square or two after dinner does the trick. Some of the chocolate bars include additions such as coconut, mint, and nuts, which reduce the glycaemic index. Similarly, if you really crave a treat like hot cocoa on a cold winter's night, try it only occasionally.

- "I have sugar cravings."

This is particularly common with stress, and in the early stages of your shift from a diet based on carbohydrates to one based on good fats. A good way to squelch sugar cravings is to take MCT oil, 1000 mg or even a teaspoon. You should avoid the standard artificial sweeteners—aspartame (sold as Canderel in UK), saccharin (pink packets of *Sweet'N Low*), and sucralose (yellow packets of *Splenda*). Stevia is a safer sweetener.

- "MCT oil and coconut oil are saturated fats—can't I try something else to help me get into mild ketosis?"

Yes, MCT oil and coconut oil are forms of saturated fat. The problem with saturated fat occurs when it is combined with sugars or other simple carbohydrates and lack of fibre. If you are keeping up your fibre intake and minimizing simple carbohydrates, then saturated fat is not usually a problem. But if you want to minimize your consumption of saturated fat, use the MCT oil for the first several weeks of the programme, since MCT helps produce the mild ketosis you're after; then switch to other forms of fats, such as extra-virgin olive oil, nuts, and avocados. That will keep your LDL particle number healthy, your small dense LDL in the healthy range, and your oxidized LDL in the healthy range. It's the best of both worlds, with mild ketosis, conversion to fat-based metabolism, and healthy lipid profile.

- "Does it matter how much water I drink? And what kind?"

It is a good idea to drink filtered water, especially for those with type 1.5 (glycotoxic) or type 3 (toxic), since pure water consumption reduces diabetes risk and helps you to excrete toxins. Shoot for about two litres per day. Herbal teas are also an excellent way to help with hydration, and the herbs described above can be included in the teas.

- "I don't have time to exercise."

Perhaps you work best with a trainer or in a class, or hiking or biking or interacting with a social network. Experiment so you find what works best for you. If time is the limiting factor, then try working it into your normal activities, such as running up your stairs or biking to work or exercising with the television at home.

- "I can't reduce stress in my life."

Take some time off, go to a spa, try meditation, use the Neural Agility programme ("meditation on steroids"), listen to music you love, take relaxing walks, enjoy the art that you love—slow down and relax!

- "This is just too complicated; I can't even keep straight what I'm supposed to do!"

I look forward to the day when there really is a simple way to address all of the many potential contributors to cognitive decline. But although ReCODE has many components, for now it's the most effective way to prevent and reverse memory loss and impaired cognition since it addresses all of the mechanisms that are *causing* the cognitive decline. That said, we are working diligently to reduce the programme's complexity—which unfortunately is dictated by the complexity of the biochemistry of cognitive decline. With further research, we should be able to be more definitive about the minimum, and the optimal, number of synapse-preserving and synapse-destroying factors that need to be addressed in each person. Until then, however, do as much of your own personalized programme as possible. As you follow up and see improvement in your lab numbers, you can begin to shed parts of the programme, as appropriate, on the advice of your practitioner or health coach. For example, many people note that, as their metabolic status improves, their hormone levels optimize naturally, so they do not need supplementation. Similarly, inflammation improves and there is no need for active anti-inflammatory treatment. You may be surprised that you may no longer need specific medicines as you optimize your metabolism—your blood pressure may come to normal naturally, your lipid profile may optimize, and your prediabetes may disappear.

- "Can't you just give me a pill?"

Sure, but it should be taken with the rest of your personalized programme. The pill will not work by itself. As I said in chapter 8, drugs—pills—are the dessert. There is little question that drugs will be extremely important in the treatment of Alzheimer's disease, and I firmly believe that the best way to test future drug candidates is to combine them with the programmatics. If you think about the "thirty-six holes in the roof" model, then drugs are designed to be a very effective patch for one hole or a few holes, and thus should perform better when the other holes are patched. However, drugs do not address the physiological underpinnings of the disease. If your brain is on the wrong side of the synapse preserving/synapse destroying balance, if it is making amyloid, then there is a reason (or, more likely, multiple reasons), so it is important to address the root problem. A single pill cannot address the many potential contributors—thus the need for a targeted, personalized programme.

- "But there is nothing better than junk food!"

Yes, junk food pits our own evolution against us, using our innate desire for sweet and high-calorie foods to induce us to eat food with low nutritive value. This is the quickest way to metabolic syndrome and multiple chronic illnesses, including cognitive decline. Perhaps the hardest part of following the ReCODE protocol is giving up foods you love: pizza, soft drinks, pancake breakfasts. But the way to parry loss is through replacement. Adopting ReCODE offers you the opportunity for new and enjoyable experiences (by the way, novelty has cognitive benefits). So if you love soft drinks (as I did), consider kombucha (which is surprisingly decent stuff), a free-range. If you crave chicken nuggets, try free-range eggs or roasted vegetables with olive oil. My personal favourite is the kitchen-sink salad, with everything from lettuce and avocados and carrots to kidney beans and boiled egg, all with vinaigrette dressing. You'll find that your palate changes when you eat fresh, whole, healthy foods. I bet you will discover a whole new set of tastes, and will find ones you love (almost?) as much as pizza.

- "But I can't eat dinner until late at night."

To make fasting the recommended 12 to 16 hours between dinner and breakfast/brunch easier, try eating a late lunch and an early evening snack.

- "I don't like to take pills."

We are working with experts to combine components so that fewer pills are needed, while still keeping the personalized, flexible combinations necessary. We are also exploring combining the vitamins and other recommended supplements in a sachet so they can be brewed into a sort of tea or stirred into plain yoghurt. For now, several of the components, such as omega-3 fatty acids and vitamin E, are in Souvenaid, a drink. Over time, more and more combinations should be available, reducing the overall pill number. For now, you can break pills or empty capsules into water or plain yoghurt, or take them with food.

- "I love meat."

No problem: although the Ketoflex 12/3 diet is plant-based, small amounts of meat and fish are fine, especially grass-fed beef, organic free-range chicken, and wild-caught SMASH fish (salmon, mackerel, anchovies, sardines, and herring).

- "What about alcohol? Can I have a glass of wine to unwind after work?"

A single glass of wine a few nights per week is fine for most people. You don't want to get to the point where the alcohol is affecting your memory, for obvious reasons, and one of the problems with wine is that it affects your insulin the way sugar does, so keeping it to a minimum is a good idea. For similar reasons, it's helpful to minimize other alcoholic drinks.

- "You don't mention smoking. I'm guessing that's a no-no, but what about vaping electronic cigarettes?"

Standard cigarettes are a risk factor for Alzheimer's disease, and the combination of vascular damage, multiple chemical exposures, and lung damage, as well as other effects, is one to avoid. Regarding vaping electronic cigarettes, the data are not in yet, but given the gravity of the prognosis if you fail to reverse cognitive decline, I recommend avoiding them, at least until more is known about their effects on cognition and Alzheimer's risk.

- "You don't say much about soy, but if I try to reduce my meat consumption, I'm going to eat tofu and other soy-based foods. Is that okay?"

You want to eat about 1 gram of protein per kilogram of your body weight, so that actually leaves you quite a bit of room to eat fish and/or free-range eggs and/or free-range chicken and/or grass-fed beef, as well as organic tofu.

- "You say that some patients who have used ReCODE successfully drink coffee in the morning. Is that okay, and if so are there any limits on caffeine?"

As described earlier in Julie's diary, coffee is fine, and in fact coffee is associated with a reduced risk of Alzheimer's disease. Too much coffee can of course make sleeping difficult and is stressful to your adrenals, so it's good to adjust to your own tolerance.

- "What about tea?"

There are many different types of tea, and these can offer a wonderful way to get your herbs, from turmeric to ashwagandha to bacopa. Also, green tea and black tea are fine while you are on the protocol.

- "Will the Ketoflex 12/3 diet put me at risk of B_{12} or iron deficiency?"

No, your labs will tell you whether you need B$_{12}$ or iron, and these will be supplemented as appropriate; furthermore, the Ketoflex 12/3 diet outlined earlier provides for animal products (for those who want to include them in their diets) that supply B$_{12}$ and iron.

- "I like to cook with high heat—will this be a problem?"

Cooking suggestions appear in chapter 8. For cooking oils, choose oils with high smoke points or that do not produce smoke at higher temperatures; good choices are avocado oil, coconut oil, butter, ghee, or animal fat.

- "Should I avoid aluminium pans?"

The aluminium theory of Alzheimer's disease has never been substantiated; that said, you'll know from your labs whether your aluminium level is high. Given what is known currently, there is no evidence that suggests that aluminium pans must be avoided.

- "Would it be better if I ate only organic?"

Yes, given a choice, eating organic foods is preferable since they lack the pesticides that may be present in nonorganic foods. Again, as mentioned earlier, "Dirty Dozen & Clean 15" is a site to guide selection priority—http://www.fullyraw.com/dirty-dozen-clean-15. It is particularly important to choose organic foods for that group. This is particularly important for those with type 3 (toxic) Alzheimer's disease.

- "If I crave something you're telling me not to have, shouldn't I listen to my body?"

Our physiological signals are indispensable and usually accurate. They tell us when we need to eat, drink, breathe, sleep, and procreate. But these same signals also tell us to prefer sugar-laden fruit juices over water, to prefer junk foods to healthy ones, and to crave simple carbohydrates late in the evening. How do you know which drives to obey and which to resist? Fortunately, it is fairly straightforward: obey those drives that are compatible with our evolution as human beings—such as eight hours of sleep, triggered by the natural light-dark cycle, and frequent movement, and resist those incompatible with our evolution, such as eating processed foods or sugar, using incandescent lights late at night, or spending hours in a chair.

There are several ways to address the cravings, such as L-glutamine 500 mg (particularly good for sugar or alcohol cravings), MCT oil (1 g or 1 teaspoon), water consumption (much of late-evening "hunger" is adequately addressed with water), and exercise.

- "I'm too busy."

The problem with chronic illnesses such as cancer and Alzheimer's disease is that symptoms begin late in the course of the illness and are mild at first. When you develop bacterial pneumonia, you feel horrible pretty quickly, so you seek treatment; but when you have a "senior moment" or two, you don't push for early evaluation and treatment. In fact, the wife of one patient who had documented Alzheimer's disease told him, "You just have the same occasional forgetfulness that we all have." Please find the time in your busy schedule, and you will allow yourself to stay productively busy for many years. The bottom line here is that you will save yourself time—years of it—if you will focus on addressing cognitive decline for several months.

There's one other crutch that my patients have found useful.

It's not a food substitute, like coconut milk ice cream for the cow's milk kind, but something that I urge them to keep reminding themselves whenever the going gets tough. Although the main "side effect" of the ReCODE protocol is better health, including improved insulin sensitivity, improved hemoglobin A1c, better lipid profile, more energy, and better mood, it is often accompanied by weight loss and a healthier body mass index. Another important side effect is finding relaxation, peace, and joy.

What brings you joy? Listening to music? Hiking beautiful trails? Time with your family? Running with your dog? Surfing? Skiing? Dancing? Playing the piano? Watching comedy? Great (healthy) food? Great sex? Whatever it is, start to work more of your joys into your life. Try new activities. The trick is to find something you truly love. Perhaps you did not have time for kayaking or dancing or biking before, but now it is going to help save your brain and your life. Once you turn the corner and find that your cognition is improving, and that you are regaining everything that is fundamental to you and your relationships, that result should bring significant additional joy in your life. And that, my patients have found, is the strongest crutch there is.

CHAPTER 12

Resistance to Change: Machiavelli Meets Feynman

It must be remembered that there is nothing more difficult to plan, more doubtful of success nor more dangerous to manage than the creation of a new system. For the initiator has the enmity of all who profit by the preservation of the old institution and merely lukewarm defenders in those who would gain by the new one.

—NICCOLÒ MACHIAVELLI

For a successful technology, reality must take precedence over public relations, for Nature cannot be fooled.

—RICHARD FEYNMAN

If you want to be liked, talk about disruption. If you want to be hated, practice it.

—R. F. LOEB

Science advances one funeral at a time.

—MAX PLANCK

GIVEN HOW OFTEN we hear that Alzheimer's disease is neither preventable nor reversible, I wouldn't be surprised if the success stories I've shared and the scientific research that underlies ReCODE have still left you sceptical. At this point, I'm well acquainted with scepticism. A few years before my first paper on the reversal of cognitive decline was published in 2014,

I received a call from a brilliant physician who had well-documented early Alzheimer's disease. He said he knew there was nothing for Alzheimer's, but if any promising trials appeared, would I let him know? I told him his call was timely, since we had a number of people who were showing good responses to ReCODE.

He didn't believe a word I said. For each part of the protocol I explained, he responded, somewhat irascibly, "There is no published evidence that this is an effective treatment for Alzheimer's disease." I tried to explain why a programmatics approach addresses the underlying pathophysiology much better than a monotherapy, and that the modest effects of individual interventions reported in studies did not preclude the possibility that combinations would be much more effective. He remained sceptical.

After enduring his scoffing for twenty minutes or so, I finally shrugged my shoulders, shook my head, and said, "Look, give me six months, and if I can't make you better, then you can go elsewhere."

"There *is* nowhere else," he shot back, sneering.

"Well, then, what do you have to lose?" I asked.

He agreed to give ReCODE a try. After three months, his wife called to tell me he was much improved, and he remains so after three years. He later told me that he had become a believer in the protocol and had started to recommend it for his own patients.

I am reminded of the 1984 film *Blood Simple*, a sharp black comedy from the Coen brothers. Everyone involved with spilling blood became simple—irrational, unthinking. The same happens when doctors, administrators, scientists, politicians, or others are exposed to a method that does not follow the standard monotherapeutic approach, producing results they were not expecting. Let me give you a small sampling of the reactions I've gotten.

One neurologist told me he would not consider using ReCODE for his patients because "I don't like shotgun approaches." Another said, "This has too many components for FDA approval." A third said his patient, who used the ReCODE protocol, had increased his Mini-Mental State Examination score from 22 to 29 (27–30 is normal), but it was "not clear" why this had happened. Yet another said, "Since I had not heard about this protocol, it must not be important." In 2011, I ran into one of the world's leading experts on Alzheimer's disease at an Alzheimer's meeting in Paris, and he asked what I was researching. When I told him I was working on the possibility that a single drug approach might not be optimal for Alzheimer's disease, he laughed, put his hand on my shoulder, and said, "Yeah, well, don't spend too much time on that!" Another Alzheimer's expert said, "I would never order those tests because I would not know how to interpret them." Yet another expert suggested that simply starting the failed drugs earlier would be the solution for Alzheimer's disease. Following one mouse study, the headlines in the press read that the university had "just cured Alzheimer's." Two foundation officials contacted me after my 2014 paper reporting the efficacy of ReCODE and suggested that the patients did not actually have Alzheimer's disease; I showed how each had been diagnosed, after which they said, "Oh, okay." A government official approached me at a meeting and said, "I read your paper, Dale. It's kinda weird . . ."

Donald Gittet, who was tasked by no less than the G8 with ridding the world of Alzheimer's disease, listened to our unprecedented results and the need for a programme that addresses all of the "thirty-six holes in the roof" of patients with Alzheimer's disease. He said, "If you can get it down to three holes, I might be interested." Wait, what? You want us to negotiate with Alzheimer's disease itself? I tried to explain the underlying processes that drive the disease, and he responded, "That sounds like science—I'm not much for science." What? This is the guy who is supposed to be saving us from Alzheimer's disease? I realized that he knew absolutely nothing about Alzheimer's disease or neuroscience—he was captaining a ship supposedly bound for the new world of Alzheimer's therapy, but had no concept of how to sail.

No one asked about efficacy! No one mentioned families without hope. Not one of the doubters asked to see or talk with any of the patients! No one mentioned that the drugs they were prescribing did not help, so anything that might would be a major step forward. No one mentioned the hundreds of failed drug trials costing billions of dollars. As quoted in the film *The Big Short*, "Truth is like poetry. And most people f&$%ing hate poetry."

The same type of "Brain Simple" responses came from people directly involved, people who actually had firsthand evidence of the effects of the protocol:

KEN, 67, HAD FAILING MEMORY, A STRONG FAMILY HISTORY of Alzheimer's disease, and was ApoE4-positive (ApoE3/4), with Alzheimer's disease documented by amyloid PET scan and fluoro-deoxyglucose PET scan. His MRI revealed that his hippocampus had atrophied so much that it was below the 20th percentile for his age.

After ten months on ReCODE, Ken was doing very well, and his repeat MRI showed a high hippocampal volume, in the 70th percentile. However, shortly after he received the MRI report, Ken received a note from the MRI centre saying that a mistake had been made: the neuroradiologist told Ken he could not believe the improvement the computer measured was correct—or real. The neuroradiologist suggested that the report be amended to indicate that the new hippocampal volume was at the 35th percentile, and the initial report revised upward to match the 35th percentile, showing no change. The neuroradiologist could not believe such an increase was possible. Ken's films were taken to another neuroradiologist for an independent reading: he concluded that the first volume was actually below the 10th percentile, and the second well over the 80th.

So as I say, disbelief, even incredulity, is something I'm all too familiar with. Let me address some of the most common sources of scepticism:

- "My doctor told me Alzheimer's is untreatable."

That is the point of this book, and our recent publications. For the first time, cognitive decline is reversible, especially in its earliest stages. Therefore, it is critical to begin the programme as early as possible.

- "I'd rather wait to do the programme until I'm more affected—I'm not that bad now."

Please don't wait! The later you start, the more difficult it is to reverse cognitive decline.

- "None of the programme components sounds like a cure."

Cognitive decline, including dementia, is a hugely complicated process, affected by dozens of factors. Targeting all of the factors that are relevant to your case in order to change the course of the illness has yielded the greatest success to date. The fact that no one of these alone is curative does not mean that a combination may not be helpful. This does not preclude the possibility that there may one day be a monotherapy that is curative; however, the complicated biology makes this unlikely, since the therapy would have to address many contributory factors.

- "Gluten is a fad. Isn't it unlikely that gluten is actually bothering me?"

I wish. Unfortunately, research from many scientists has overturned the now outdated concept that only patients with celiac disease need worry about gluten. Gluten can compromise the integrity of the gut barrier (and potentially the blood-brain barrier), leading to leaky gut, systemic inflammation, and increasing risk for cognitive decline.

- "Some of the labs you are suggesting are not reimbursed by my insurance."

The standard evaluation for cognitive decline does not include the very tests that determine *why* it is occurring, let alone tell you how to optimize treatment. Many people are finding that their insurers will indeed cover some or most of the tests. This, of course, may not be the case in the UK. But few investments are more worthwhile than keeping yourself or a loved one out of a nursing home, which is itself extremely expensive.

- "Why haven't I heard about this? And why hasn't my doctor?"

Although my laboratory colleagues and I have published on the underlying research for ReCODE since 1993, my first paper describing patients on ReCODE appeared only in 2014, and as I write this in 2017 there have been only three additional peer-reviewed publications (one on therapeutics and two on diagnostics). Any new approach is likely to be met with scepticism—and to be ignored by much of the medical establishment—unless and until there is a large-scale, controlled clinical trial. I explained in chapter 5 why that has not yet happened, but in 2017 we are starting a proof-of-concept trial, to pave the way for a larger, first-of-its-kind clinical trial for the comprehensive ReCODE protocol.

- "Does this programme work for other causes of cognitive decline, such as Lewy body dementia, vascular dementia, multiple sclerosis, Parkinson's, and frontotemporal degeneration?"

This is an important question, but we do not yet have an answer. ReCODE was designed to address the mechanisms that drive the process of cognitive decline that causes Alzheimer's disease, and to address as many as possible of these mechanisms. As it happens, however, many of the same problems (insulin resistance, leaky gut, biotoxins, and more) that contribute to Alzheimer's disease also affect type 2 diabetes, metabolic syndrome, and cardiovascular disease. It is possible that non-Alzheimer's neurodegenerative diseases like Lewy body disease share some mechanisms. In the first few Lewy body patients who were evaluated with the tests described in chapter 7, the results resembled those in type 3 (toxin-related) Alzheimer's disease. Perhaps addressing the source of those toxins would help in Lewy body disease, too, but that research remains to be done.

- "But my lab values are normal."

"Normal values" are not necessarily good enough when you are trying to reverse cognitive decline. Lab values should be optimal, not just "within normal limits." (See chapter 8 for the details.)

- "But I already eat healthy food."

That is a great start. Let's get the rest of the programme activated in a way that is personalized for your lab values, and make sure your diet is indeed optimized for cognition.

- "I need to vent—my family and I are so frustrated, angry, and depressed. Why did this happen to me?"

You have every right to be frustrated, angry, and depressed. But cognitive decline does not occur for no reason, and the underlying causes (often a dozen or more contributors) can be identified, quantified, and addressed. It's fine to vent, but it's better to be evaluated and get going on treatment.

- "I heard that supplements and herbs are unregulated, and mostly rubbish."

Some supplements and herbs are not as advertised—some bottles don't even contain what the label claims—so it is critical to get the right ones. A top-flight herbalist, for whom I have great respect, recommends supplements and herbs from Banyan, Gaia Herbs, Metagenics, or Natura Health Products, which tend to be reliable.

- "I am not getting better—your protocol must not work!"

Troubleshooting with your practitioner or health coach can pinpoint the problem. Here are some possibilities:

1. How long have you been on the protocol? It takes three to six months to see initial improvement. Reversing years of damage does not happen overnight.

2. How well documented is the problem? Might you have something other than this Alzheimer's-related SCI or MCI? It is important to rule out multiple strokes and alcohol-related cognitive decline, for instance, since ReCODE was not designed for those disorders.

3. If you have been following the optimal protocol for at least six months, and your lab values have improved but your cognition has not, something has been missed. You do not suffer cognitive decline for no reason, so it is important to continue to evaluate and tweak your protocol. For instance, have you induced mild ketosis? Have you changed from a carbohydrate-based diet to a good fats-based one? A very common sign that the metabolism has changed is a reduction in weight, typically of 4.5 to 18 kg depending on your starting weight. Also, as noted above, the best responses occur early in the process of cognitive decline. If you have moderate Alzheimer's, improvement is unfortunately more difficult.

4. The most common cause of a failure to respond is failing to truly follow the programme. The second most common cause is having type 3 (toxic) Alzheimer's, which requires additional steps to eliminate the exposure and treat the effects of the toxin. If you have features of type 3, seek an expert in chronic inflammatory response syndrome (CIRS), such as those listed at survivingmold.com.

5. Another common problem is undiagnosed sleep apnea. Has this been ruled out? And are you getting at least seven hours of sleep each night?

6. Are you doing the brain training for thirty minutes per day, three times per week, or ten to twenty minutes per day five times per week? If so, have you truly seen continued decline on your cognitive tests, despite this training? Or are you improving, but not at the rate you had hoped? The first

change that should occur is a cessation of decline, followed by very modest improvement—for example, getting better at something you could not previously do, such as remember passages you had read or follow directions.

7. Have your labs reached the optimal values, as outlined in the table in chapter 7?

ReCODE has now worked for hundreds of people. So even if you have a genetic risk for Alzheimer's, are already suffering from subjective or mild cognitive impairment, or have been diagnosed with early Alzheimer's itself, take a deep breath and shed the hopeless, helpless feeling. It often helps to talk with someone who has improved on the protocol, so it does not feel like some sort of fantasy or empty promise. Then decide whether you really want to fight cognitive decline with this protocol. No one and nothing can help you if you do not want to be better.

I described in chapter 5 what it's like to go up against powerful corporations and closed-minded experts who can't tolerate any deviation from the reigning paradigm—even when that paradigm has failed as abysmally as it has in Alzheimer's disease. Fortunately, one of the great things about science is that evidence trumps everything else—at least eventually.

The only way to evaluate the efficacy of a medical treatment is by ascertaining whether it helps people improve. Not does it bring in funding, not does it make money, not does it get published in a sexy journal, not does it garner approbation from colleagues, not does it bring accolades, but does it help people to improve? This seems simple and obvious, but in reality it is a surprisingly rare priority. This "cognition compass" is especially important in Alzheimer's disease because there is currently no alternative. It's not as if there are multiple effective therapeutics and we are simply trying to improve on them. To the contrary, the current standard of care has nothing that stops, let alone reverses, the cognitive decline in subjective cognitive impairment, mild cognitive impairment, or Alzheimer's disease.

Part of the problem is that the stakes are too high and the bar is too low. With a trillion-dollar global problem—for that's what Alzheimer's disease is—the temptation is just too great, and this brings out the liars, the bottom-feeders, the snake-oil salesmen, and the like. For instance, even as experts tell me they don't believe our published, peer-reviewed results, imitators are starting companies that purport to offer the same protocol, even though they have no expertise in the field and no knowledge of the current protocols. One company was started by a businesswoman and a few pathologists; when they were told that their protocol was out-of-date, the response was "It's good enough to make money." Another imitator was started by a couple of unethical computer IT guys, who have no expertise in medicine, let alone neurology. If your printer is jammed, these guys may be helpful, but if you are concerned about cognition, you'll want to consult a doctor, preferably one who understands the underlying problem. Sadly, these sorts of companies are trafficking in human desperation.

The trillion-dollar temptation is just too great. When this kind of money is at stake, objectivity is eclipsed: as they say, "The big picture tends to be obscured by the a$$ you are kissing."

Make no mistake, changing the fundamentals of the Alzheimer's world will create a stentorian conflagration, a collective frictional cringe. The goal of reducing the global burden of dementia will always be at risk of getting lost in the scramble for sales, for grants, for tenure, for prizes, for political gain, for fund-raising.

Christian Bale, playing Dr. Michael Burry in the film *The Big Short*, said that "rather than following numbers or facts, people choose to follow that which seems authoritative and familiar." This can have disastrous consequences, just as it did in the financial meltdown that began in 2008. Nearly 200 years ago, Dr. Ignaz Semmelweis was able to save the lives of countless new mothers by realizing that their high rate of postpartum mortality must be due to the transfer of pathogens from the cadavers the medical students worked on before helping to deliver babies. He determined that this could be almost completely prevented through washing hands with a solution of calcium hypochlorite. Because the whole concept of infectious illnesses was not understood at that time, the experts did not believe Semmelweis. One authority argued that "it seems improbable that enough infective matter or vapor could be secluded around the fingernails to kill a patient." Ultimately, the medical leaders forced Semmelweis to be committed to an insane asylum where he was beaten and, ironically, died from a resulting infection.

As we continue to evolve and improve the approach to preventing and reversing cognitive decline, we will need open minds—for outside-the-box trials, new types of tests and data sets, and global prevention programmes. Developing a true cure for Alzheimer's disease requires that our experts and leaders be sharper and more open-minded than those of Semmelweis's era.

For centuries, we humans typically died from acute infections such as bacterial pneumonia, and the great biomedical success of the twentieth century was to develop antibiotics that treat them and public health policies that prevent them. As a result, most of us now die from chronic, complex illnesses such as cancer, cardiovascular disease, and neurodegenerative disorders. Unfortunately, we tried to solve the problem of chronic illness in the same way we solved the problem of acute illness: with a single pill, monotherapy. This is like using your draughts strategy in a chess match.

Let me repeat something I said in chapter 1: *No one should die from Alzheimer's disease.* I hope that, no matter how sceptical you were when you read that the first time, I have persuaded you that it is not only possible in theory but within our reach today. To make the end of Alzheimer's reality for everyone, however, will require that we update our practices from twentieth-century medicine to twenty-first-century medicine, and that we be proactive about our own cognitive and general health. It will require that we follow our own personalized, optimal health programme. This is completely different from twentieth-century healthcare. No longer will people wait for symptoms to appear to see a practitioner, especially as the realization takes hold that although symptoms are relatively early manifestations of acute illnesses (think of how quickly your nose starts to run or your throat starts to ache when you get an upper respiratory tract infection), they are late manifestations of chronic illnesses. With twenty-first-century medicine, people will no longer await the onset of symptoms before making targeted changes in their lives to address a chronic illness; they will manage their health, using an individualized approach such as ReCODE, throughout life.

To achieve twenty-first-century medicine, we will have to close the complexity gap, the chasm between the tremendous complexity of the human organism and the rudimentary data on which we now base diagnostic and therapeutic decisions. Checking your sodium and potassium won't show why you developed Alzheimer's disease.

Imagine that you are trying to learn to fly an airplane, but your instructor tells you that you have no altimeter, no airspeed indicator, and an opaque windshield; the only data you have will be from a thermometer that tells you the temperature of the left wingtip. You would crash pretty much every time, right? Well, that is what is happening with chronic illnesses such as Alzheimer's disease. We check things like sodium and potassium, and we fail to check the parameters that are driving the illness.

We must therefore close this complexity gap by gathering key data that match the complexities of our minds and bodies. Only then can we hope to prevent and reverse Alzheimer's disease.

With twenty-first-century medicine, diagnoses will not be guesswork and will be more complete. For example, instead of a twentieth-century diagnosis of subjective cognitive impairment, the twenty-first-century diagnosis may be subjective cognitive impairment of types 1.5 (70 per cent) and 3 (30 per cent), due to grade 3 central insulin resistance, AGE-associated autoantibodies, and innate immune system activation due to *Aspergillus* and HLA-DR/DQ 12-3-52B interaction, with associated gliotoxin production. The treatment would then be a personalized protocol that addresses all of these contributors.

Closing the complexity gap will change everything. It will let us see chronic illnesses coming decades before they strike, and will also prevent them. Closing the complexity gap will let doctors determine quickly whether prevention or treatment is working, allowing clinicians to get their patients back on course to good health and the avoidance of serious disorders. Diagnosis will no longer be a guessing game. And it will be feasible to reduce the global burden of dementia dramatically, reduce health care costs by hundreds of billions of dollars, improve decision-making, and enhance longevity.

Closing the complexity gap will create twenty-first-century healthcare, and with it a world without the dread of dementia, a world without families destroyed by cognitive loss. As they say, a goal is a dream with a deadline. Working together, we can realize these dreams.

"Everyone knows a cancer survivor, but no one knows an Alzheimer's survivor." As I hope I have succeeded in showing you in this book, that is yesterday's news. The world has changed.

Appendices

Appendix A

Summary of Foods to Eat and Foods to Avoid

Let me break down for you what I call red light, yellow light, and green light foods: those to avoid at all costs, those it's okay to have in moderation (largely because avoiding them entirely makes Re-CODE too difficult to follow for many people—the "some is better than none" principle), and those you can indulge in to your heart's content.

Foods to eat frequently, less frequently, or avoid altogether.

Green light foods: eat frequently	Yellow light foods: eat less frequently	Red light foods: avoid if possible
Mushrooms	Starchy vegetables such as potatoes (sweet potatoes are an exception; see below), corn, peas, and squash	Sugar and other simple carbohydrates, including bread (white and whole meal), pasta, rice, biscuits, cakes, sweets, fizzy drinks
Cruciferous vegetables such as broccoli, cauliflower, and Brussels sprouts	Legumes such as peas and beans	Grains
Leafy green vegetables such as kale, spinach, and lettuce	Nightshades such as aubergines, peppers, and tomatoes	Gluten

Green light foods: eat frequently	Yellow light foods: eat less frequently	Red light foods: avoid if possible
Wild-caught fish, especially SMASH fish (salmon, mackerel, anchovies, sardines, and herring)	Nontropical fruits—fruits with low glycaemic indices, such as berries	Dairy—minimize, but occasional cheese or organic whole milk (or raw milk) or plain yoghurt is all right
Free-range eggs	Free-range chicken	Processed foods (if it's in a package with ingredients listed, avoid)
Resistant starches such as sweet potatoes, swedes, parsnips, and green bananas	Grass-fed beef	High-mercury fish such as tuna, shark, and swordfish
Probiotic foods such as sauerkraut and kimchi	Wine (limit to one glass a few times per week)	Fruits with high glycaemic indices, such as pineapple
Prebiotic foods such as jicama (Mexican yam) and leeks	Coffee	
Herbal tea, black tea, green tea		
Sulphur-containing vegetables such as onions and garlic		

Functional medicine practitioners:

https://www.functionalmedicine.org/practitioner_search
.aspx?id=117

Health and wellness coaches:

http://www.findahealthcoach.com/

Information on CIRS (chronic inflammatory response syndrome):

http://www.survivingmold.com/

Direct to consumer laboratory testing:
    https://www.anylabtestnow.com/
    https://www.aacc.org/~/media/files/position-statements/
        directtoconsumerlaboratorytesting2.pdf?la=en

ApoE4 support and discussion:
    www.apoe4.info

Additional information:
    https://www.drbredesen.com
    https://www.mpicognition.com

Appendix B

Ketone Meter Details

- The Ketostix (urine) testing is too imprecise to be helpful for most people.
- One example is the Precision Xtra meter, which determines both glucose and ketones. The glucose strips are quite affordable. The ketone strips are pricier, and Julie Gregory from the website ApoE4.info suggests purchasing them from Canada, since they are more affordable.
- No prescription is needed for a ketone meter.
- The meter costs about £27; here is one site for purchasing the ketone meter: https://www.amazon.com. Type in "precision glucose ketone monitoring system."
- The goal is to keep beta-hydroxybutyrate from 0.5 mmol/L to 4 mmol/L, which indicates mild ketosis.
- After you have used the ketone meter to determine when you are in mild ketosis, you won't have to use this every day or even every week or month, since you will have an idea about what it takes to make you mildly ketotic, and of course the meter will still be available for you to check any time.

Appendix C

Having DNA from 23andMe Evaluated

Note that 23andMe does not provide a full genome, and therefore not all SNPs (single nucleotide polymorphisms, which are DNA differences) associated with Alzheimer's disease will be evaluated. However, ApoE status should be reported (about 85 per cent of the time, ApoE status will be reported), and 23andMe has just restarted their reporting of ApoE status.

Ordering your kit

- On the web, go to 23andme.com and click on the "how it works" tab.
- Click on the "shop now" button.
- Select "Health + Ancestry and click on the "add to cart" button to begin setting up your profile and credit card billing. Be sure to remember the user ID and password for your new account.
- When you receive the DNA kit in the post, open it and follow the instructions inside.
- Visit 23andMe and select "register kit."
- Post the sample back to 23andMe.

- You will receive a confirmation email from 23andMe once your sample reaches their lab.

Accessing your genome file

You will receive an email from 23andMe when your genome sequencing has been completed.

1. Log in to your account on the 23andMe website to download your genome data.
2. Click on your profile name at the top right, after logging in.
3. Select: BROWSE RAW DATA.
4. On their next webpage, click on the "Download" button.
5. Specify the Profile to download (yours).
6. Choose "All DNA."
7. Verify you've downloaded a file whose zipped size is about 5 MB to 30 MB. The downloaded file's name is of the form: Genome_*Your_Name*_Full_*date*.zip.

Once you have received this file, it can be analyzed by websites such as Promethease (https://www.promethease.com/).

Appendix D

For those who wonder what is the basis for our approach to the ReCODE protocol, I have provided a thumbnail below. Additional information is available in our over 200 peer-reviewed publications, many of which are freely available online.

Proof of the Theory Behind ReCODE Programmatics

Tenet	Evidence
There exists a plasticity balance that affects memory storage vs. reorganization/forgetting.	Eidetic memory; D664A mutants; alterations
APP is a mediator of the plasticity balance.	D664A mutant[1]
The 4:2 ratio reflects the APP-mediated plasticity balance.	D664A mutant;[2] ApoE4 effect; inflammatory effect
Alzheimer's (AD) risk factors such as ApoE4 alter the plasticity balance, and alter the 4:2 ratio.	[3]
APP is a dependence receptor.	[4,5,6]
The probability of developing ADα [synaptoclastic signalling]/ [synaptoblastic signalling]	Transgenics; human APP mutants; epidemiology
APP functions as a molecular switch.	Inhibitory effects of sAPPα, αCTF, and amyloid-beta
APP-Aβ form a prionic loop.	[7]

Tenet	Evidence
The origin of prions is in biological signal amplification.	Anti-homeostatic signalling in systems requiring amplification and featuring multigoal outcomes.
Aggregation modulates signalling.	Homomeric activating complexes such as caspases.[8]
AD is a neurodegenerative plasticity imbalance due to a protective response to metabolic, infectious/inflammatory, or toxic inducers.	Epidemiology; NF-κB response;[9]; type 3 patients; mercury effects
A treatment for SCI, MCI, and AD involves shifting the plasticity balance toward synaptoblastic signalling and away from synaptoclastic signalling.	[10,11]

Explanation for the proof:

- There exists a plasticity balance that affects memory storage vs. reorganization/forgetting. The phenomenon of eidetic memory (photographic memory) supports this point, and further evidence is provided by manipulating this balance. The mutation of the caspase site in APP reduces the memory-loss effect of "Mouzheimer's disease" transgenic mice. Conversely, introducing Alzheimer's-associated mutations in APP into the mice causes the memory loss associated with "Mouzheimer's." Introducing the mutation that improves the "Mouzheimer's mice" into a normal mouse actually improves its retention of memory. All of these findings support the tenet that there is a plasticity balance that affects memory storage vs. reorganization/forgetting.

- APP is a mediator of the plasticity balance. As noted above, mutations of APP—at the beta site, gamma site, and caspase site, for example—alter this balance in both directions, in a predictable way—both toward better memory and toward worse memory. These findings support the tenet that APP itself is a mediator of the plasticity balance.

- The 4:2 ratio reflects the APP-mediated plasticity balance. Mutations and other manipulations, such as trophic factor additions, that increase the 4 APP-derived peptides sAPPβ, Aβ, Jcasp, and C31, or reduce the two APP-derived peptides sAPPα and αCTF, reduce memory performance and increase the Alzheimer's pathophysiological changes. Conversely, mutations and other manipulations that decrease this same ratio have the opposing effect, improving memory performance and decreasing Alzheimer's-associated pathophysiological changes.

- AD risk factors such as ApoE4 alter the plasticity balance, and alter the 4:2 ratio. Risk factors such as ApoE4, reduced oestrogen, reduced vitamin D, and many others, all increase this 4:2 ratio, and conversely, risk reducers such as exercise and BDNF all reduce this same ratio.

- APP is a dependence receptor. As demonstrated in the references listed in the table above, APP displays the features of a dependence receptor, such as a single intracellular caspase site and binding to a trophic factor—here, netrin-1.

- The probability of developing AD α [synaptoclastic signaling]/[synaptoblastic signalling]. Just as occurs with osteoclastic vs. osteoblastic signalling in osteoporosis, the probability of developing Alzheimer's disease is proportional to the ratio of the synaptoclastic signalling vs. the synaptoblastic signalling, and modulating this ratio in either direction exerts the predicted effect on risk of disease and on progression vs. regression of the disease. This tenet is supported by many familial Alzheimer's disease mutations, all of which increase this ratio, as well as by the many epidemiological risk factors and inhibitors, from exercise to hormones to trophic support.

- APP functions as a molecular switch. The derivatives of APP cleavage feed back to inhibit the alternative cleavage pathway—for example, CTFα inhibits the gamma-site cleavage—and therefore, the cleavage path tends toward one direction or another, functioning as a switch.

- APP-Aβ form a prionic loop. As a corollary to the tenet immediately above, the addition of amyloid-beta to APP increases the generation of amyloid-beta, as demonstrated in the reference cited in the table. Thus APP and Aβ form a prionic loop, with the amyloid-beta causing more amyloid-beta to be generated from APP, which feeds back to increase the process.

- The origin of prions is in biological signal amplification. Systems such as blood clotting, in which rapid amplification is required and the outcome is not a single goal—whether this is thrombus vs. nonthrombotic state or neurite extension vs. retraction, etc.—feature anti-homeostatic signalling, and thus the mediators beget more of themselves or their signalling. These are the features of prions.

- Aggregation modulates signalling. As shown in many systems, the self-interaction (homomeric interaction) of proteins is often involved in specific effects such as activation. In some caspases, for example, aggregation leads to rapid activation.

- AD is a neurodegenerative plasticity imbalance due to a protective response to metabolic, infectious/inflammatory, or toxic inducers. As noted in the text, the shift of APP processing toward the four pro-Alzheimer's peptides, which is the path that produces the amyloid, is a protective response to three major metabolic or toxic perturbations: inflammation, trophic withdrawal, or toxic exposure. This protective response is associated with a downsizing of the synaptic network.

- A treatment for SCI, MCI, and AD involves shifting the plasticity balance toward synaptoblastic signalling and away from synaptoclastic signalling. The final proof of the theory is provided by the finding that humans (not just mice or other animal models) with SCI, MCI, or early AD have shown improvement following a shift of the balance toward synaptoblastic signalling, as described in the references cited.

Acknowledgements

HOW DOES ONE go about trying to develop an effective treatment for an incurable illness? One that has proven resistant to hundreds of drug candidates? Little can be done without the support of truly remarkable and caring individuals. I am grateful beyond what I can express here to Jim and Phyllis Easton for their generosity and friendship, and for ensuring that Mary's illness would not be in vain; to Dr. Patrick Soon-Shiong for his remarkable vision; to Douglas and Ellen Rosenberg for taking a risk; to Beryl Buck, Dagmar and David Dolby; Stephen D. Bechtel Jr.; Diana Merriam and the Four Winds Foundation; Gayle Brown; Diana Chambers; Katherine Gehl; Larry and Gunnel Dingus; Michaela Hoag; Lucinda Watson; Tom Marshall and the Joseph Drown Foundation; Jeffrey Lipton; Wright Robinson; and Shar McBee.

I have had the great privilege of learning from some of the foremost scientists and doctors in the world, and I am grateful for their unparalleled instruction and tutelage. My most sincere thanks go to Professors Stanley Prusiner, Mark Wrighton (Chancellor), Roger Sperry, Robert Collins, Robert Fishman, Roger Simon, Vishwanath Lingappa, William Schwartz, Kenneth McCarty Jr., J. Richard Baringer, Neil Raskin, Robert Layzer,

Seymour Benzer, Erkki Ruoslahti, Lee Hood, and Mike Merzenich.

I am also grateful to the functional medicine pioneers and experts who are revolutionizing medicine and who are my respected colleagues: Drs. Jeffrey Bland, David Perlmutter, Mark Hyman, Dean Ornish, Ritchie Shoemaker, Sara Gottfried, David Jones, Patrick Hanaway, Terry Wahls, Stephen Gundry, Ari Vojdani, Tom O'Bryan, Nathan Price, Jared Roach, and Chris Kresser, among others; and social network activists Julie Gregory and her colleagues from the ApoE4.info website, as well as to courageous individuals like Patient Zero, Deborah Sonnenberg, and David B. who are, through their discipline and hard work, helping so many others with cognitive decline. Thanks also go to doctors who cared for or consulted on some of the patients described in this book, including Drs. Mary Kay Ross, Edwin Amos, Ann Hathaway, Kathleen Toups, Rangan Chatterjee, Ayan Panja, Susan Sklar, Carol Diamond, Ritchie Shoemaker, Mary Ackerley, Sunjya Schweig, Raj Patel, Sharon Hausman-Cohen, Nate Bergman, Kim Clawson Rosenstein, Wes Youngberg, Karen Koffler, Craig Tanio, Dave Jenkins, health coach Amylee Amos, Aarti Batavia, and the hundreds of doctors from seven countries and around the United States who have participated in, and contributed to, the course focused on the protocol described in this book. In addition, I am grateful to Lance Kelly and his group at Apollo Health, and Juan Porras and his group at Factivate, for their outstanding work on the ReCODE algorithm, coding, and reports.

None of what is described in this book would have been possible without the outstanding laboratory members and colleagues with whom I have worked over the past three decades. For the fascinating discussions, the many whiteboard sessions, the countless hours of experimentation, the patience to repeat and repeat experiments, and the unflagging dedication to enhancing humankind's health and knowledge, I am grateful to Shahrooz Rabizadeh, Patrick Mehlen, Varghese John, Rammohan Rao, Patricia Spilman, Rowena Abulencia, Kayvan Niazi, Litao Zhong, Alexei Kurakin, Veronica Galvan, Darci Kane, Karen Poksay, Clare Peters-Libeu, Veena Theendakara, Alex Matalis, and all of the other present and past members of the Bredesen Laboratory, as well as to my colleagues at the Buck Institute for Research on Aging, UCSF, the Sanford Burnham Prebys Medical Discovery Institute, and UCLA.

For their friendship and many discussions over the years, I thank Thom Mount, Leigha Hodnet, Shahrooz Rabizadeh, Patrick Mehlen, Dan Lowenstein, Bruce Miller, Stephen Hauser, Mike Ellerby, David Greenberg, John Reed, Guy Salvesen, Tuck Finch, Nuria Assa-Munt, Kim and Rob Rosenstein, Eric and Carol Adolfson, Judy and Paul Bernstein, Beverly and Roldan Boorman, Sandy and Harlan Kleiman, Philip Bredesen and Andrea Conte, Deborah Freeman, Peter Logan, Sandi and Bill Nicholson, Stephen and Mary Kay Ross, Raj Ratan, Mary McEachron, and Douglas Green.

Finally, I am grateful for the outstanding team with which I have worked on this book: for the writing and editing of Sharon Begley, Dedi Felman, and Thom Mount; literary agents John Maas and Celeste Fine of Sterling Lord Literistic; and editor Caroline Sutton, publisher Megan Newman, and Avery Books at Penguin Random House.

Notes

Chapter 4: How to Give Yourself Alzheimer's: A Primer

1. Kumar, D. K., *et al.* Amyloid-beta peptide protects against microbial infection in mouse and worm models of Alzheimer's disease. *Science Translational Medicine* 8: 340ra72, doi: 10.1126/scitranslmed.aaf1059 (2016).
2. Kumar, D. K., W. A. Eimer, R. E. Tanzi, and R. D. Moir. Alzheimer's disease: the potential therapeutic role of the natural antibiotic amyloid-beta peptide. *Neurodegenerative Disease Management* 6: 345–348, doi: 10.2217/nmt-2016-0035 (2016).

Chapter 5: Wit's End: From Bedside to Bench and Back

1. https://en.wikipedia.org/wiki/Dependence_receptor.
2. Lourenço, F. C., *et al.* Netrin-1 interacts with amyloid precursor protein and regulates amyloid-beta production. *Cell Death and Differentiation* 16: 655–663, doi: cdd2008191 [pii]10.1038/cdd.2008.191 (2009).
3. Galvan, V., et al. Reversal of Alzheimer's-like pathology and behavior in human APP transgenic mice by mutation of Asp664. *Proceedings of the National Academy of Science USA* 103: 7130–7135, doi: 10.1073/pnas.0509695103 (2006).
4. Spilman, P., *et al.* The multi-functional drug tropisetron binds APP and normalizes cognition in a murine Alzheimer's model. *Brain Research* 1551: 25–44, doi: 10.1016/j.brainres.2013.12.029 (2014).
5. Ibid.
6. Clarkson, T. W., L. Magos, and G. J. Myers. The toxicology of mercury— current exposures and clinical manifestations. *New England Journal of Medicine* 349: 1731–1737, doi: 10.1056/NEJMra022471 (2003).

Chapter 6: The God Gene and the Three Types of Alzheimer's Disease

1. Mutter, J., A. Curth, J. Naumann, R. Deth, and H. Walach. Does inorganic mercury play a role in Alzheimer's disease? A systematic review and an integrated molecular mechanism. *Journal of Alzheimer's Disease* 22: 357–374, doi:10.3233/JAD-2010-100705 (2010).

Chapter 7: The "Cognoscopy"—Where Do You Stand?

1. den Heijer, T., *et al.* Homocysteine and brain atrophy on MRI of non-demented elderly. *Brain* 126 (Pt 1): 170–175 (2003).
2. Rocca, W. A., B. R. Grossardt, L. T. Shuster, and E. A. Stewart. Hysterectomy, oophorectomy, estrogen, and the risk of dementia. *Neurodegenerative Diseases* 10: 175–178, doi: 10.1159/000334764 (2012).
3. Brewer, G. J. Copper excess, zinc deficiency, and cognition loss in Alzheimer's disease. *Biofactors* 38: 107–113, doi: 10.1002/biof.1005 (2012).
4. Chausmer, A. B. Zinc, insulin and diabetes. *Journal of the American College of Nutrition* 17: 109–115 (1998).
5. Liu, G., J. G. Weinger, Z. L. Lu, F. Xue, and S. Sadeghpour. Efficacy and safety of MMFS-01, a synapse density enhancer, for treating cognitive impairment in older adults: a randomized, double-blind, placebo-controlled trial. *Journal of Alzheimer's Disease* 49: 971–990, doi: 10.3233/JAD-150538 (2016).
6. Smorgon, C., *et al.* Trace elements and cognitive impairment: an elderly cohort study. *Archives of Gerontology and Geriatrics Supplement* 9: 393–402, doi: 10.1016/j.archger.2004.04.050 (2004).
7. Tyler, C. R., and A. M. Allan. The effects of arsenic exposure on neurological and cognitive dysfunction in human and rodent studies: a review. *Current Environmental Health Reports* 132–147, Report No. 2196-5412 (Electronic) (2014).
8. Basha, M. R., *et al.* The fetal basis of amyloidogenesis: exposure to lead and latent overexpression of amyloid precursor protein and beta-amyloid in the aging brain. *Journal of Neuroscience* 25: 823–829, doi: 10.1523/JNEU-ROSCI.4335-04.2005 (2005).
9. Bakulski, K. M., L. S. Rozek, D. C. Dolinoy, H. L. Paulson, and H. Hu. Alzheimer's disease and environmental exposure to lead: the epidemiologic evidence and potential role of epigenetics. *Current Alzheimer Research* 9: 563–573 (2012).
10. Ashok A., N. K. Rai, S. Tripathi, and S. Bandyopadhyay. Exposure to As-, Cd-, and Pb-mixture induces Aβ, amyloidogenic APP processing and cognitive impairments via oxidative stress-dependent neuroinflammation in young rats. *Toxicological Sciences* 143: 64–80, doi: 10.1093/toxsci/kfu208 (2015).

11. Dysken, M. W. *et al.* Effect of vitamin E and memantine on functional decline in Alzheimer disease: the TEAM-AD VA cooperative randomized trial. *Journal of the American Medical Association* 311: 33–44, doi: 10.1001/jama.2013.282834 (2014).

12. Poole, S., S. K. Singhrao, L. Kesavalu, M. A. Curtis, and S. Crean. Determining the presence of periodontopathic virulence factors in short-term postmortem Alzheimer's disease brain tissue. *Journal of Alzheimer's Disease 36:* 665–677, doi: 10.3233/JAD-121918 (2013).

13. Descamps, O., Q. Zhang, V. John, and D. E. Bredesen. Induction of the C-terminal proteolytic cleavage of AβPP by statins. *Journal of Alzheimer's Disease* 25: 51–57, doi: 10.3233/JAD-2011-101857 (2011).

14. Bredesen, D. E. Inhalational Alzheimer's disease: an unrecognized—and treatable—epidemic. *Aging (Albany NY)* 8: 304–313 (2016).

Chapter 8: ReCODE: Reversing Cognitive Decline

1. Heijer, T., *et al.* Association between blood pressure levels over time and brain atrophy in the elderly. *Neurobiology of Aging* 24: 307–313 (2003).

2. http://www.health.harvard.edu/diseases-and-conditions/glycemic-index -and-glycemic-load-for-100-foods.

3. Khan, A., M. Safdar, M. M. Ali Khan, K. N. Khattak, and R. A. Anderson. Cinnamon improves glucose and lipids of people with type 2 diabetes. *Diabetes Care* 26: 3215–3218 (2003).

4. http://articles.mercola.com/sites/articles/archive/2014/09/21/hilary -boynton-mary-brackett-gaps-cookbook-interview.aspx.

5. https://draxe.com/scd-diet/

6. http://www.drperlmutter.com/learn/resources/probiotics-five-core -species.

7. Thrasher, J. D., M. R. Gray, K. H. Kilburn, D. P. Dennis, and A. Yu. A water-damaged home and health of occupants: a case study. *Journal of Environmental and Public Health* 2012, doi: 10.1155/2012/312836 (2012).

8. http://www.survivingmold.com/shoemaker-protocol/Certified -Physicians-Shoemaker-Protocol

9. https://www.functionalmedicine.org/practitioner_search.aspx?id=117.

10. Shoemaker, R. C., MD. *Surviving Mold: Life in the Era of Dangerous Buildings.* Otter Bay Books, 2010.

Appendix D

1. Galvan, V., *et al.* Reversal of Alzheimer's-like pathology and behavior in human APP transgenic mice by mutation of Asp664. *Proceedings of the National Academy of Science USA* 103: 7130–7135, doi:10.1073/pnas.0509695103 (2006).

2. *Ibid.*

3. Theendakara, V., et al. Neuroprotective sirtuin ratio reversed by ApoE4. *Proceedings of the National Academy of Science USA* 110: 18303–18308, doi: 10.1073/pnas.1314145110 (2013).

4. Lourenço, F. C., *et al.* Netrin-1 interacts with amyloid precursor protein and regulates amyloid-beta production. *Cell Death and Differentiation* 16: 655–663, doi: cdd2008191 [pii]10.1038/cdd.2008.191 (2009).

5. Lu, D. C., *et al.* A second cytotoxic proteolytic peptide derived from amyloid-beta-protein precursor. *Nature Medicine* 6: 397–404, doi:10.1038/74656 (2000).

6. Spilman, P., B. Jagodzinska, D. E. Bredesen, and John Varghese. Enhancement of sAPPα as a therapeutic strategy for Alzheimer's and other neurodegenerative diseases. *HSOA Journal of Alzheimer's & Neurodegenerative Diseases* 1: 1–10 (2015).

7. Spilman, P. R., et al. Netrin-1 interrupts amyloid-beta amplification, increases sAβPPα in vitro and in vivo, and improves cognition in a mouse model of Alzheimer's disease. *Journal of Alzheimer's Disease* 52: 223–242, doi: 10.3233/JAD-151046 (2016).

8. Julien, O., *et al.* Unraveling the mechanism of cell death induced by chemical fibrils. *Nature Chemical Biology* 10: 969–976, doi: 10.1038/nchembio.1639 (2014).

9. Matrone, C., *et al.* Activation of the amyloidogenic route by NGF deprivation induces apoptotic death in PC12 cells. *Journal of Alzheimer's Disease* 13: 81–96 (2008).

10. Bredesen, D. E. Reversal of cognitive decline: A novel therapeutic program. *Aging* 6: 707–717, doi: 10.18632/aging.100690 (2014).

11. Bredesen, D. E., *et al.* Reversal of cognitive decline in Alzheimer's disease. *Aging* 8: 1250–1258, doi: 10.18632/aging.100981 (2016).

Index